Doga

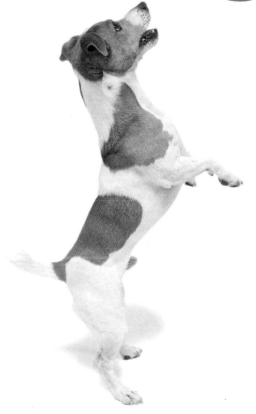

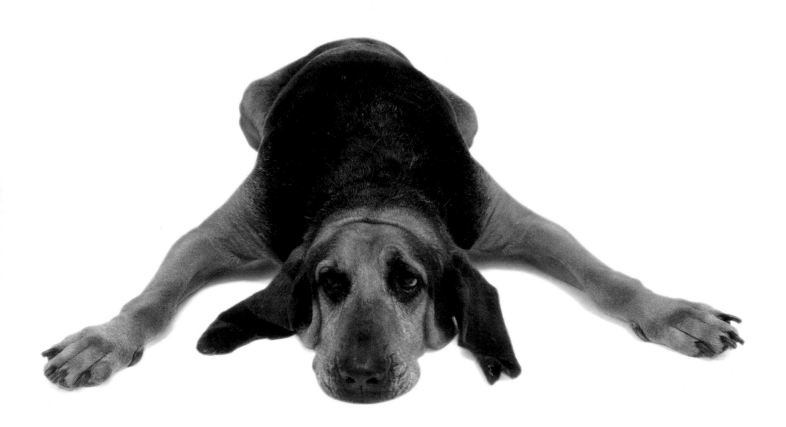

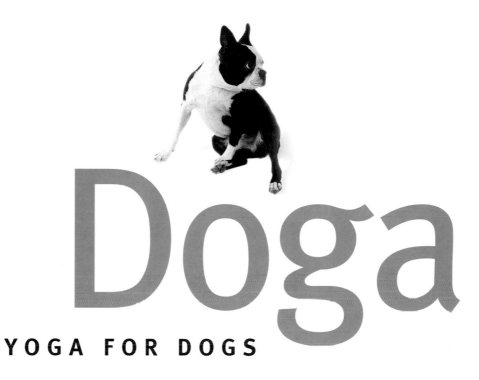

Doga

YOGA FOR DOGS

By Jennifer Brilliant

And William Berloni, Animal Consultant

With Bennie, Buster, Cricket, Harlem, Kessie, and Pi

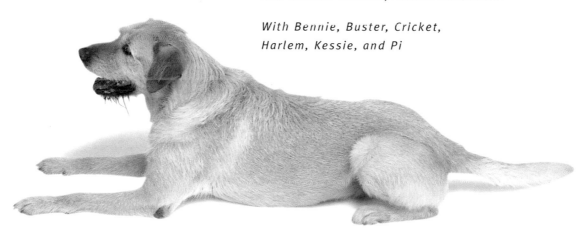

CHRONICLE BOOKS

SAN FRANCISCO

Library of Congress Cataloging-in-Publication Data:

Brilliant, Jennifer.
  Doga : yoga for dogs / by Jennifer Brilliant and William Berloni.
    p. cm.
  ISBN 0-8118-4167-7
  1. Dogs—Exercise. 2. Yoga. I. Berloni, William. II. Title.
  SF427.45.B75 2003
  636.7'08937046—dc21

                        2003008012

Printed in China

A Quirk Packaging Production
Editorial direction by Sharyn Rosart
Cover design by Lynne Yeamans and Julie Vermeer
Interior design by Lynne Yeamans

Distributed in Canada by Raincoast Books
9050 Shaughnessy Street
Vancouver, British Columbia V6P 6E5

10 9 8 7 6 5 4 3 2 1

Chronicle Books LLC
85 Second Street
San Francisco, California 94105

www.chroniclebooks.com

**The authors and publisher would like to stress that the dogs in
this book, and dogs in general, do these positions naturally. At
no time were the dogs forced into any poses, and you should
not attempt to force or otherwise coerce your dog into any of
the positions in this book or any other yoga-based positions.
Follow the principles of yoga, let your dog do what comes naturally, and enjoy what you can learn from observing. Namaste.**

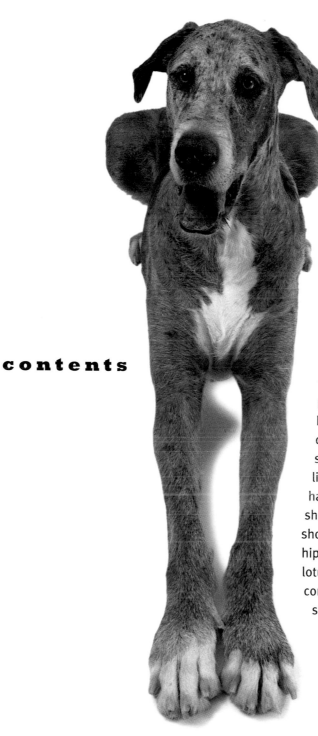

contents

introduction

As long as dogs have walked the earth they have practiced doga (pronounced DOH-gah). Doga is no secret: anyone who has spent time around a dog has probably witnessed the ancient practice of doga. Many humans, however, would not recognize doga, but merely assume that the dog was scratching a persistent itch or thinking about dinner.

What is doga? In general, doga is best thought of as a philosophy of living that helps its practitioners to unite body and mind in healthy, joyous awareness. One who practices doga is called a dogi (DOH-ghee).

In the past to receive the teachings of doga, it was necessary to sit at the paws of a practicing dogi, and to carefully study the dogi's actions. Most human knowledge of doga came from this kind of devoted study, which led eventually to the development of what humans call yoga. Now, however, for the first time, several master dogis have come together to share their knowledge and experience in a way that can be easily translated for human students. At last, the wisdom of doga is readily available through these pages.

We can learn about our own humanity by studying doga. Simply being with a dogi can be enlightening.

"Doga is a journey, an exploration of our bodies and minds—a cultivation of awareness, for example of moving into, being in, and moving out of naps, and savoring each step along the way."

—Kessie

"Doga is a way of life, not something separate from life. Doga is retrieving a stick; doga is digging a hole; doga is greeting another dogi with a good, long sniff."

—Cricket

6

"Doga is an ancient process designed to help you uncover and discover your true nature so you can live daily life, take daily walks, and enjoy daily naps with that awareness."

—Buster

"Doga is for everyone. Since ancient times, doga has been continuously adapted to suit the needs of individuals from different species, cultures, and traditions. All who come are welcome."

—Harlem

A dogi's commitment to living in the moment helps us to be more aware of the mystery and magic of life present in our everyday tasks. Taking loving care of a dogi companion is a spiritual practice in itself.

Doga teaches us even more. When we see dogis practicing doga, we see their true nature. We are inspired to relax like they do and be ourselves. Dogis are able to accept themselves exactly as they are in each moment. This is a valuable life lesson.

Dogis never make comparisons between themselves and other dogis. They do not care that another dogi has bigger paws or a smaller butt, or can hold downward-facing dog for a longer period. They are never compelled to push themselves further into a pose. They follow their breath and respect their bodies.

Dogis accept themselves and the world around them. They revel in the smells and tastes of living, giving themselves over fully to each new sensation. Dogis often attempt to show their human companions the joys of fully accepting experience—inviting us to roll in a cool mud puddle or to sniff at a delicious-smelling morsel on the street. While we may not indulge in those particular pleasures, this joyful acceptance is also something we can learn from them.

Dogis never try to impress. They practice doga with effortlessness and compassion, self-aware but never self-conscious.

Though there can be obstacles along the path of doga, such as laziness or boredom, dogis rarely become frustrated or deviate from the path. Dogis know that their practice takes time and they develop patience. Occasionally a dogi is distracted from the practice— squirrels, treats, and unexpected visitors can disturb their concentration. But they have the commitment to simply start back up again with eagerness. They are con-tinually in the present moment. They show us that fantastic moments of great insight may arise during seemingly mundane tasks such as grooming one's paws.

Over the centuries since humans first adapted yoga from doga, the practice has changed and been adapted for human anatomy and human nature, but the original lessons remain to be learned. If you practice yoga, you may have already realized that you can learn from dogis, simply by observing their downward- and upward-facing dog poses. This book will help you open your mind to the full benefits of doga, bringing its lessons to your entire practice.

"It is not necessary to be already 'fit' to do doga. The key is to accept and use your body as it is at the present moment. Use all your sensations to make an inquiry into yourself. Who are you? What are your favorite smells?"

—Pi

"Doga is the path that cultivates the body and senses, refines the mind, lifts the tail, and brings ease to the soul."

—Bennie

meet the dogis

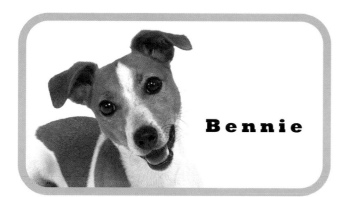 Bennie

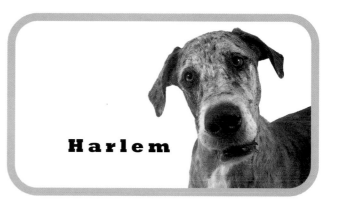 Harlem

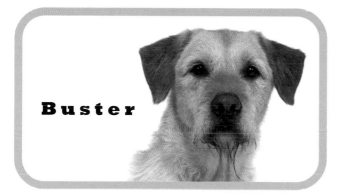 Buster

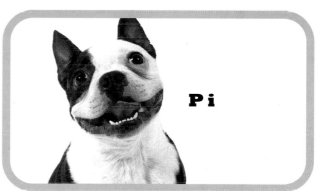 Pi

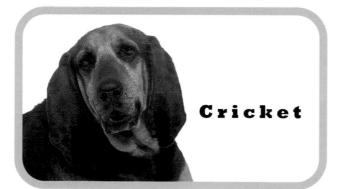 Cricket

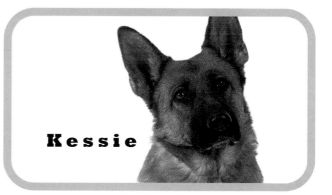 Kessie

opening chants

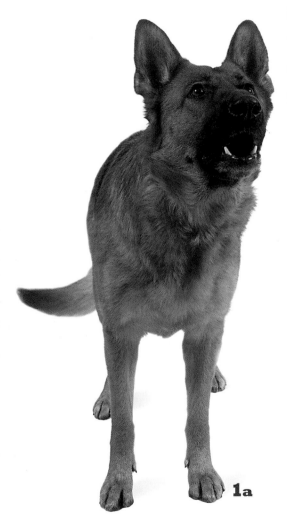

Dogis find that chanting is an excellent way to open the practice of doga. The most common opening chant is the repetition of **OM**. An ancient syllable with many meanings, om is often described as the original sound, the first vibration of energy. When many dogis chant together, the sound is often described as "howling," but to dogis it is the sound of the universe.

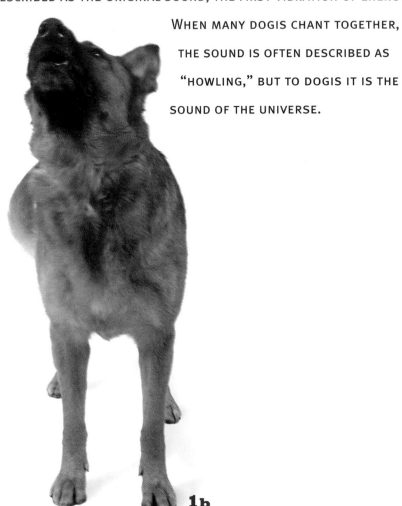

1a

1b

1a To begin her chanting, Kessie first takes a firm, well-grounded stance. Note how her paws are pressing into the ground, her head is lifted, and her chest is open to allow the free and full movement of her breath from her belly up through her throat. She draws in a deep inhalation in preparation for her om.

1b Kessie demonstrates how the syllable om can be chanted by enunciating the separate sounds of **a**—"ah," **u**—"ooh," and **m**—"mmm."

2 After Kessie has chanted om three times, each time feeling the vibration move through her body, she feels strong and inwardly focused. Now she is ready to begin her practice.

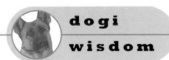

dogi wisdom

"Everyone, dogis and yogis and even cats, has a 'third eye,' the spot right between the eyebrows. That's where to focus during chanting." —Kessie

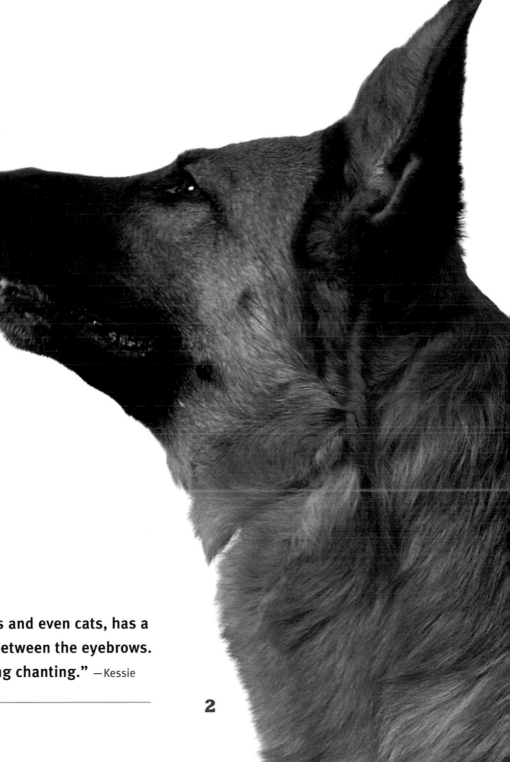

breathing awareness

DOGA PRACTICE BEGINS WITH BREATHING. **PRANAYAMA** (*PRANA* MEANS "VITAL ENERGY OF LIFE," THAT IS, BREATH, WHILE *YAMA* MEANS "CONTROL" OR "MASTERY") IS THE PRACTICE OF GAINING CONTROL OVER THE BREATH. DOGIS HAVE MASTERED MANY BREATHING TECHNIQUES; ALL BEGIN WITH SIMPLE AWARENESS.

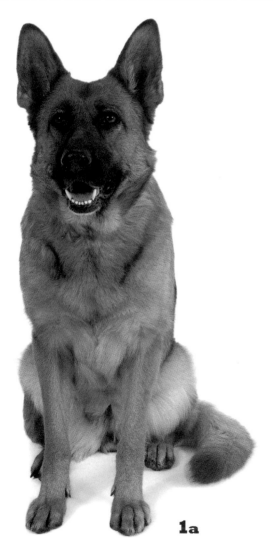

1a

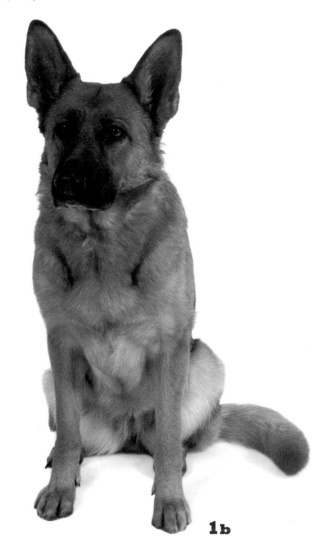

1b

1a Kessie sits with her back elongated, chest open, and flanks firmly settled on the floor. A good seated posture is essential to the practice of pranayama. Kessie begins to observe her breaths, noting their natural rhythm and sound.

1b Kessie deliberately slows her breathing, controlling her inhalations and exhalations. She gently closes her jaws, and breathes through her nose only.

2 Pi demonstrates the benefits of breath control. His oxygen intake has increased, enhancing the functioning of all his bodily systems. His back lengthens and his chest expands to take in even more air. As he focuses inward, his gaze softens.

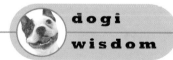

dogi wisdom

"During breathing awareness, I sometimes give a little snort to clear my nasal passages. Regular breathing practice is excellent for the sinuses." —Pi

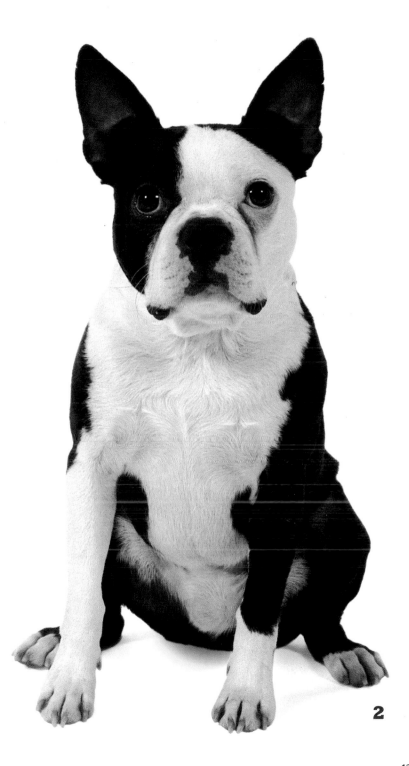

2

victorious breath

UJJAYI (YU-JYE-EE), OR VICTORIOUS, BREATHING IS
AN INTEGRAL PART OF ALL DOGA PRACTICE, DONE
ON ITS OWN AND DURING THE ASANAS. UJJAYI
ALSO MEANS "TO CONQUER"; AS THE DOGI FILLS HIS
LUNGS, HIS CHEST SWELLS LIKE THAT OF A CONQUEROR.

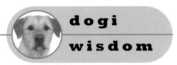

dogi wisdom

**"Make a sound that's something between
a growl and a purr."** —Buster

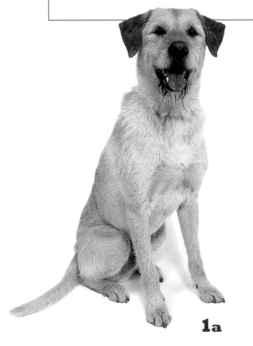

1a

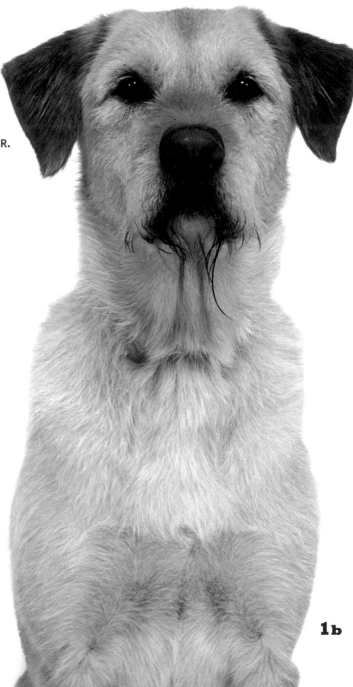

1b

1a Buster gets ready to begin his ujjayi breathing by taking a regal posture with a firmly grounded seat.

1b Buster closes his mouth and draws in air through his nose. He consciously narrows his throat, slightly constricting the passageway for the breath, so as to have more control over it. He maintains this control through inhalation and exhalation. The narrowing of the throat creates the characteristic sound of ujjayi, a sound that may be likened to a soft roar. Note the openness of Buster's nostrils to maximize the flow of air.

2 Bennie's mastery of ujjayi breathing is so profound that he can control the vibration of his whiskers as he breathes.

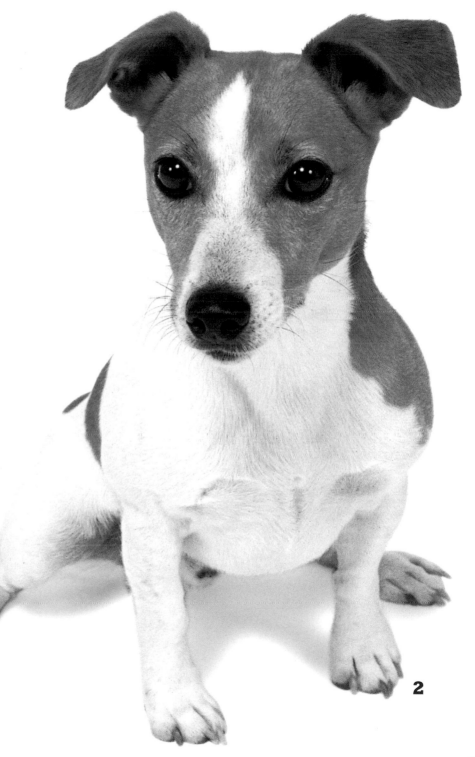

2

chin lock

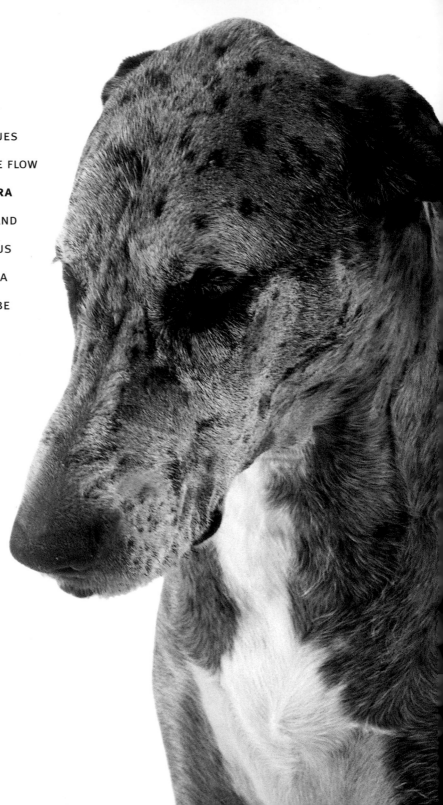

Locks, or **BANDHAS**, are advanced techniques that dogis use to control and contain the flow of breath energy. The chin lock, **JALANDHARA BANDHA** (jahl-an-DAR-ah BAHN-da), calms and contains the energy generated by vigorous breathing. The concentrated stillness of a dogi controlling her energy should not be confused with resting.

To perform a chin lock, the dogi pauses consciously at the end of the indrawn breath, gently holding the breath for a few seconds. Similarly, at the end of the exhalation, the dogi rests briefly without breathing, calm and serene. To engage her chin lock, Harlem draws her chin down towards her chest while simultaneously lifting her chest up towards her chin.

breath of fire

BREATH OF FIRE (ALSO KNOWN AS "HOT BREATH" OR "PANTING") IS A CLEANSING, STIMULATING BREATH. AN ACTIVE BREATHING TECHNIQUE, IT USES THE BODY'S OWN HEAT ENERGY (DOGIS CAN TRANSFER HEAT THROUGH THEIR TONGUES). IN BREATH OF FIRE, INHALATION AND EXHALATION ARE FORCEFUL: THE BREATH IS EXHALED WITH A STRONG CONTRACTION OF THE ABDOMINAL MUSCLES, FOLLOWED BY A FAST, VIGOROUS INHALATION.

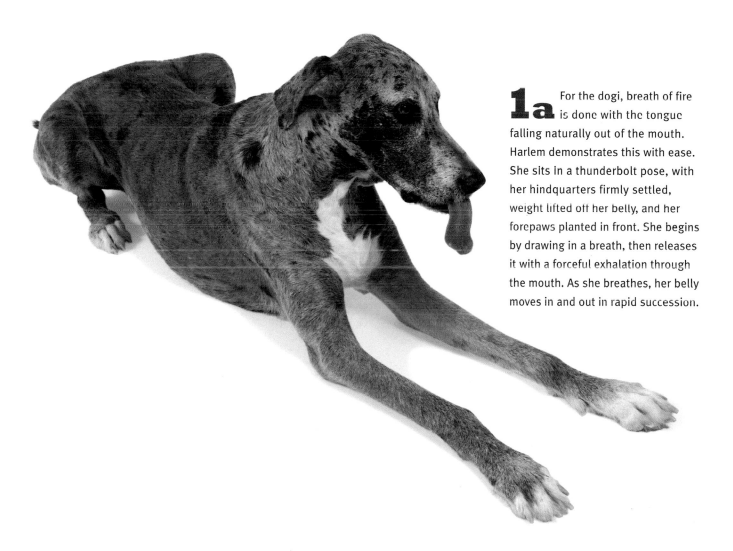

1a For the dogi, breath of fire is done with the tongue falling naturally out of the mouth. Harlem demonstrates this with ease. She sits in a thunderbolt pose, with her hindquarters firmly settled, weight lifted off her belly, and her forepaws planted in front. She begins by drawing in a breath, then releases it with a forceful exhalation through the mouth. As she breathes, her belly moves in and out in rapid succession.

1b Breath of fire is also a cleansing breath, which means that there is often drool or drainage from the sinuses. One advantage that dogis have over human practitioners is their ability to easily sweep away any waste products with a quick swipe of the tongue. Harlem swiftly cleans up between cycles.

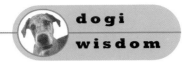

dogi wisdom

"Though breath of fire does not necessarily mean that I am thirsty, a bowl of fresh, cool water is always nice to have." —Harlem

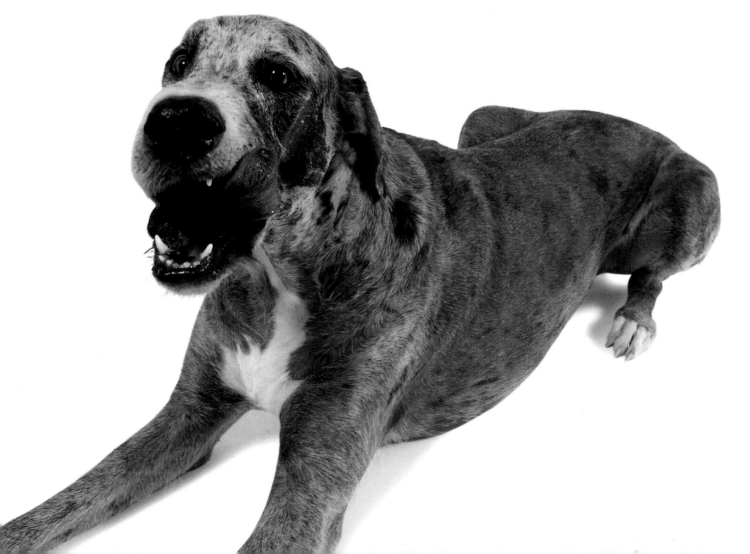

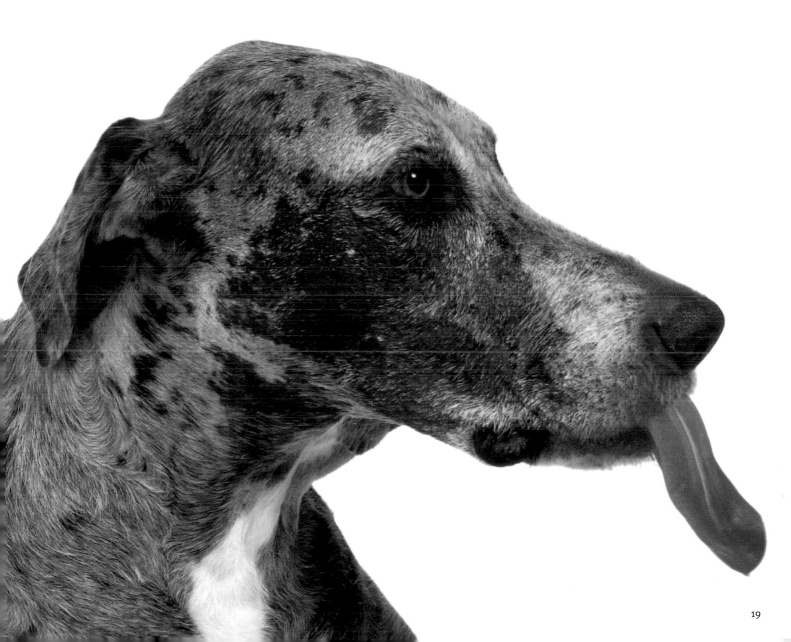

2 After one round of 10 to 15 breaths, Harlem rests briefly, closing her mouth and breathing normally, before extruding her tongue to begin another cycle.

alternate-nostril breathing

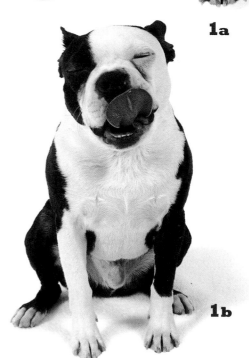

NADI SHODHANA (NAH-DEE SHO-DAH-NAH), OR ALTERNATE-NOSTRIL BREATHING, IS A BREATH-CONTROL TECHNIQUE THAT REQUIRES INHALING AND EXHALING THROUGH A SINGLE NOSTRIL. IT IS ESPECIALLY GOOD FOR DOGIS (AND HUMANS) WHO SUFFER FROM NASAL CONGESTION OR STUFFINESS.

1a

1a To begin, Pi extends his tongue and uses it to close off the right nostril. Then he inhales slowly through the left nostril and fills his lungs. After a complete inhalation, he presses the left nostril closed with his tongue, and opening the right nostril, exhales slowly.

1b After a complete exhalation, Pi inhales through the right nostril and fills his lungs. He then extrudes his tongue, and closes off the right nostril. After opening the left nostril, he breathes out slowly. This process is one round of nadi shodhana.

1b

cooling breath

ANOTHER OF THE ACTIVE PRANAYAMAS OFTEN PRACTICED BY DOGIS
IS **SITALI** (SEE-TAH-LEE), OR "CURVED BEAK" BREATH. THIS IS A
BREATH THAT IS USED WHEN THE DOGI FEELS OVERHEATED, BECAUSE
OF ITS ABILITY TO COOL AND SOOTHE THE BODY AND MIND. SITALI
BREATH IS CHARACTERIZED BY A HISSING SOUND, WHICH HUMANS
OFTEN MISTAKE FOR SIGHING.

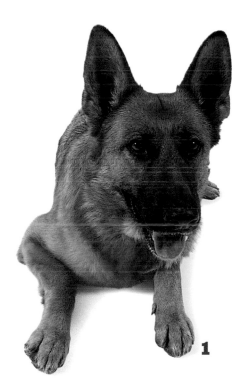

1 Kessie extrudes her tongue very slightly, while curling the side edges upward (inside the teeth), creating a long tube. She then draws in a breath through this tube. As the air passes through her curled tongue, Kessie feels cooler. As she exhales, she releases the hotter, stinkier air through her nostrils.

2 One of the most important aspects of doga is the attitude with which it is practiced. Note the lightness of spirit that Pi brings to his practice. In his cooling breath, the corners of his mouth upturn in a slight smile. Keeping an inner smile is actually a practice in itself.

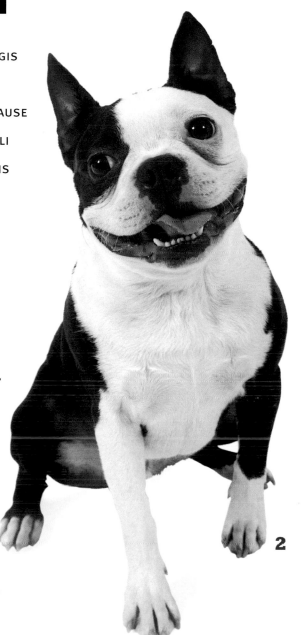

mountain pose

Having achieved a calm yet alert state through their breathing practice, the dogis are ready for standing poses. The first of these is **TADASANA** (TAH-DAHSS-anna), or mountain pose. Tadasana is the beginning and end of all standing poses.

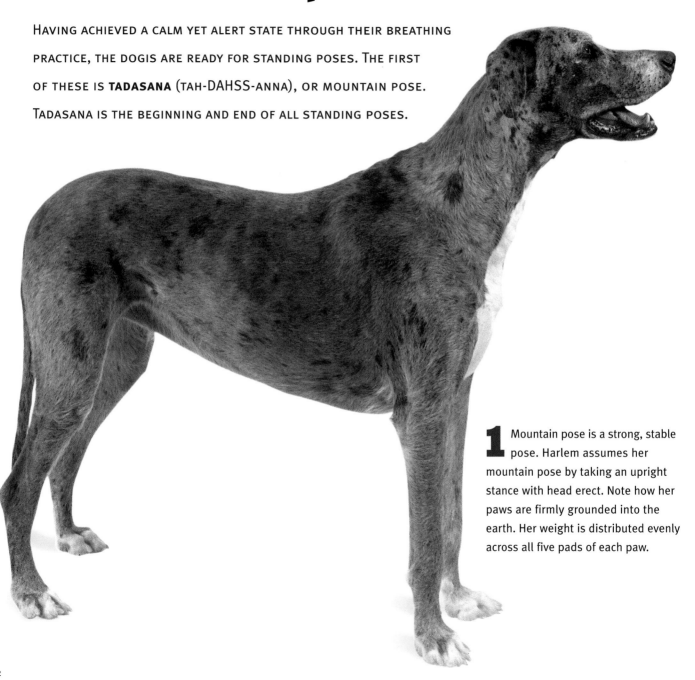

1 Mountain pose is a strong, stable pose. Harlem assumes her mountain pose by taking an upright stance with head erect. Note how her paws are firmly grounded into the earth. Her weight is distributed evenly across all five pads of each paw.

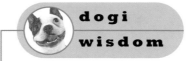
"In tadasana, I sometimes visualize myself as a mountain, with other mountains standing tall around me. Sometimes they are mountains of kibble; I practice restraint, observing my desire to eat but not acting on it." —Pi

2 As Pi presses his paws firmly downward, his upper body and head lift. Though his gaze remains soft, Pi's concentration demonstrates an intense connection to the earth. In the union of opposites that creates balance in doga, a firmly grounded stance gives Pi a paradoxical lightness.

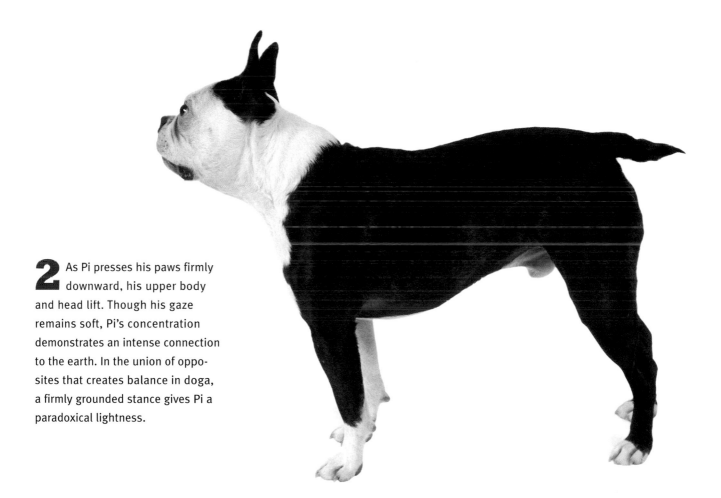

downward-facing dog

ONE OF THE BEST-KNOWN DOGA POSES, DOWNWARD-FACING DOG, OR **ADHO MUKHA SVANASANA** (AH-doh MOO-kuh shvah-NAHSS-anna), IS AN INTEGRAL PART OF ALL DOGA PRACTICE. EMPHASIZING THE DOGA PRINCIPLE OF OPPOSITES, DOWNWARD-FACING DOG REQUIRES THE DOGI TO PRESS DOWNWARD AND STRETCH UPWARD AT ONCE. THIS POSE ALSO SAYS "PLAY-WITH-ME," A MESSAGE THAT INSPIRED THE FIRST YOGIS TO GET DOWN AND IMITATE THEIR DOGIS.

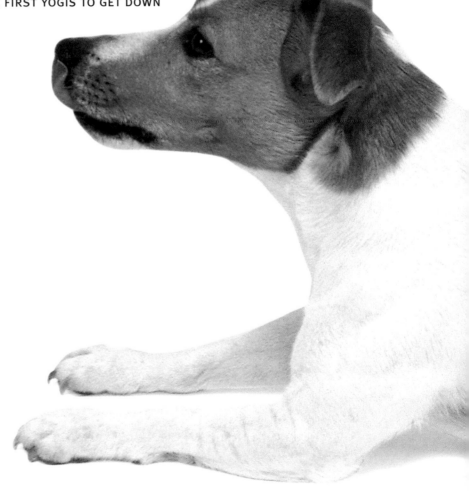

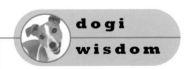 **dogi wisdom**

"For extra stretch, lift your tail to the sky! If you don't have one, imagine that you do." —Bennie

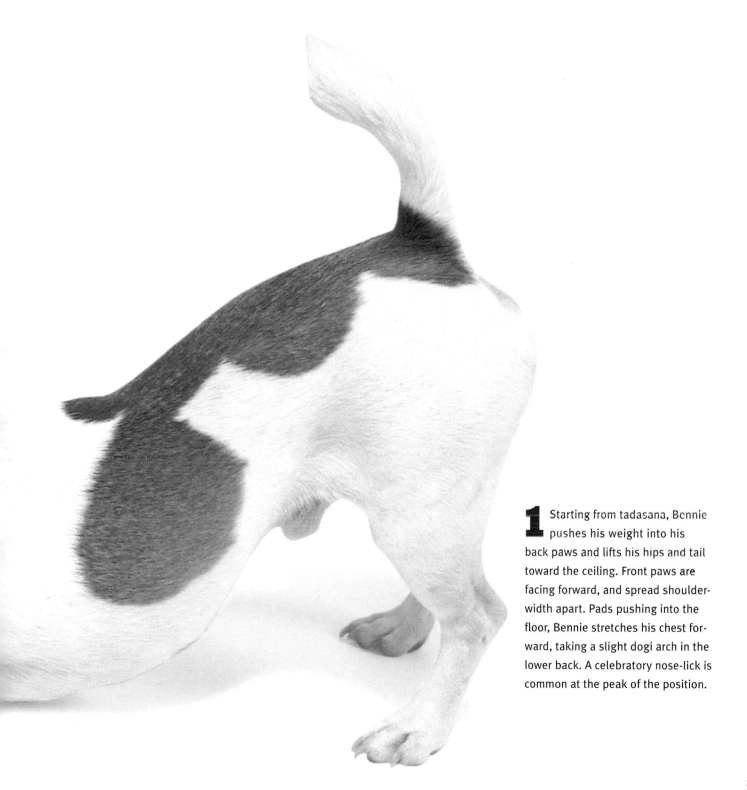

1 Starting from tadasana, Bennie pushes his weight into his back paws and lifts his hips and tail toward the ceiling. Front paws are facing forward, and spread shoulder-width apart. Pads pushing into the floor, Bennie stretches his chest forward, taking a slight dogi arch in the lower back. A celebratory nose-lick is common at the peak of the position.

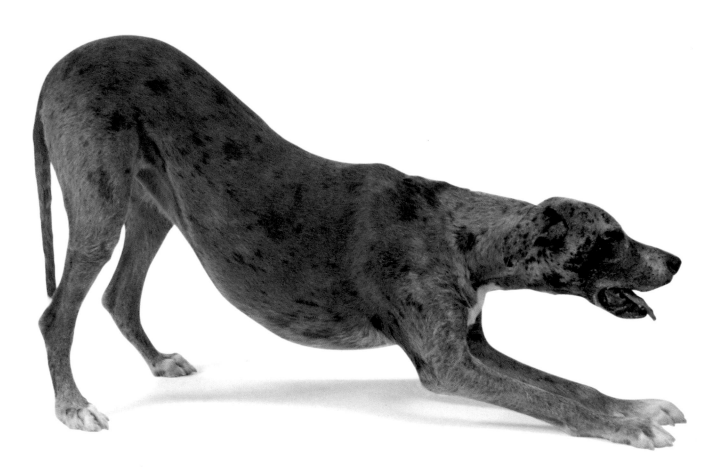

2a Downward-facing dog is a favorite pose of many dogis. This pose has so many benefits that it is easy to see why all dogis do it. They love downward-facing dog for the stretch it gives their leg muscles, which tend to get tight from chasing squirrels. It is also an excellent position from which to greet another dogi with a long, respectful sniff.

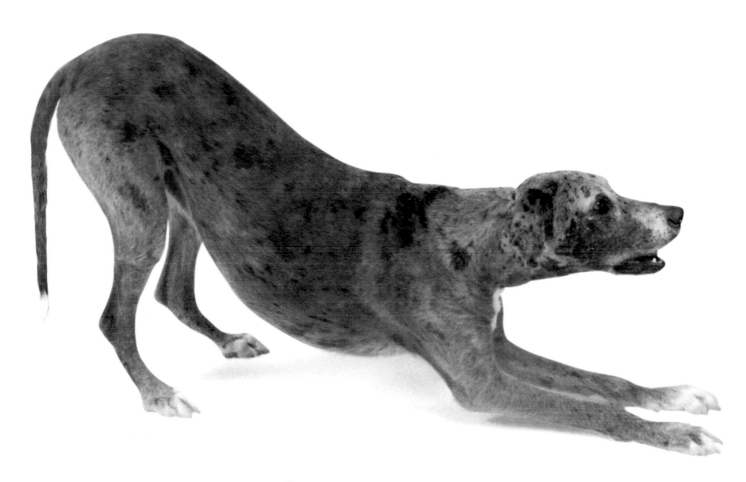

2b Downward-facing dog can relieve compression along the spinal cord. It feels like a big yawn for the whole dogi. To deepen her pose, Harlem pushes her haunches back even farther, tail down for balance, and lifts her head. She is ready to spring into action, especially if someone throws a ball.

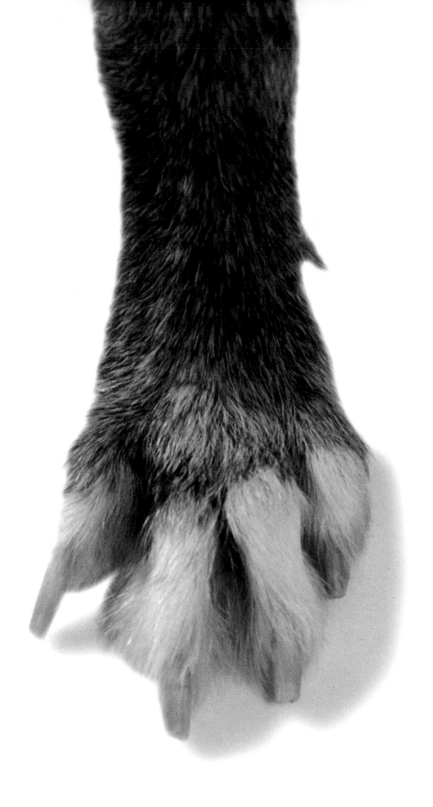

3 Because the paws are the points of contact with the · earth from which the dogi draws strength, paw position is particularly important in downward-facing dog. Each of the pads is in full contact with the floor. Harlem presses her pads evenly into the ground, so there is no strain anywhere in the paw. There is an equal amount of distance between each toe. Harlem thinks of the space between each toe like a gateway for her bounding energy.

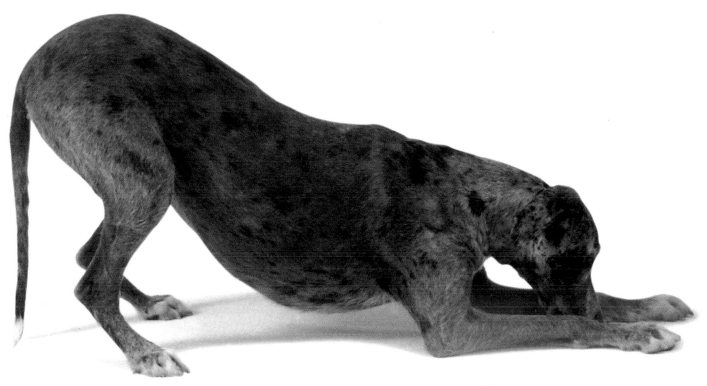

4 Downward-facing dog is a challenging pose, which requires both strength and flexibility. If the dogi begins to feel overwhelmed, downward-facing dog can also be done as a restorative pose by placing the head and/or elbows on the floor. Harlem demonstrates this variation, which is also useful if the dogi is fatigued, and wishes to transition to a lying-down pose.

upward-facing dog

Upward-facing dog, **URDHVA MUKHA SVANASANA** (OOHRD-va MOO-kah shvah-NASS-anna), is another fundamental doga pose. An invigorating pose, upward-facing dog aligns the spine and invigorates the kidneys (a walk may be needed soon after practicing this asana).

1 Anyone who observes a dogi with any frequency will see the dogi performing this asana. Dogis naturally do upward-facing dog for the benefits it gives as a counterpose to long periods of meditative contemplation (not to be mistaken as lying around).

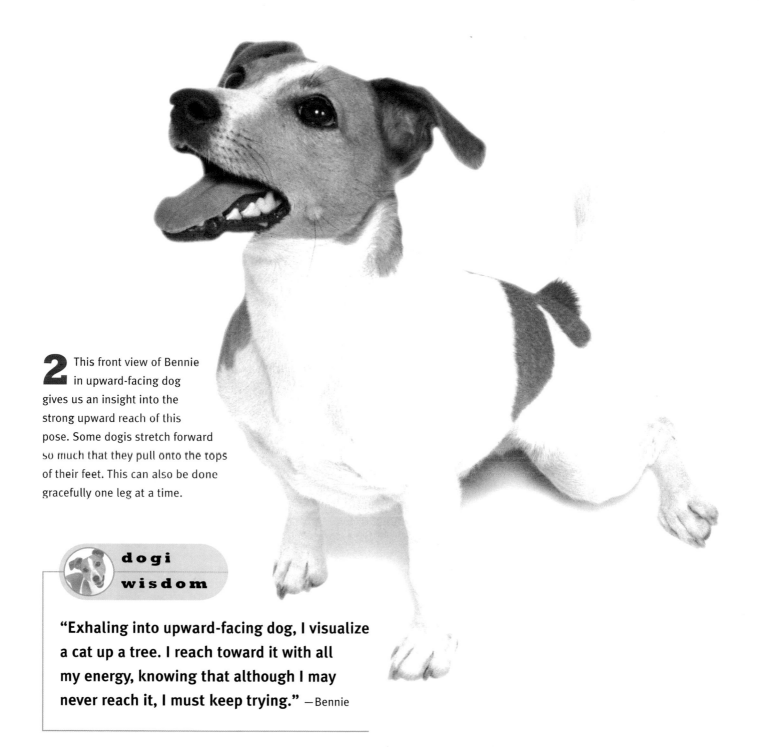

2 This front view of Bennie in upward-facing dog gives us an insight into the strong upward reach of this pose. Some dogis stretch forward so much that they pull onto the tops of their feet. This can also be done gracefully one leg at a time.

dogi wisdom

"Exhaling into upward-facing dog, I visualize a cat up a tree. I reach toward it with all my energy, knowing that although I may never reach it, I must keep trying." —Bennie

upward-paw pose

The Sun Salutation, or **SURYA NAMASKAR** (SOO-REE-AH NAHM-AHSS-CAR), IS A SERIES OF POSES THAT DOGIS DO TO GREET EACH DAY. IT INCORPORATES FORWARD AND BACKWARD BENDS TO CREATE THE OPTIMUM BALANCE OF STRENGTH AND FLEXIBILITY. THE SUN SALUTATION BEGINS WITH THE UPWARD-PAW POSE, OR **URDHVA HASTASANA** (OORD-VAH HAHSS-TAHSS-ANNA). MOST DOGIS SALUTE THE SUN DAILY.

1 Standing firmly on the earth that supports him, Bennie reaches his paws upward to the sun. He lifts his head to the sky, keeping his back upright. He gratefully receives the sunlight into his heart with deep peace. He feels warm and refreshed.

human tip

With no tail to help balance them, yogis should keep their tailbones down (but not tucked).

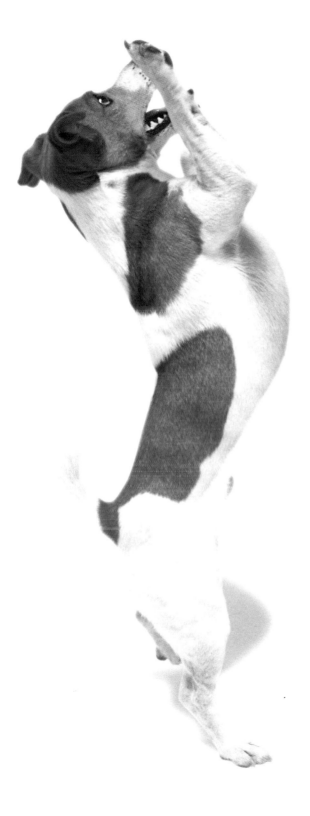

2 Inhaling, Bennie extends his stretch and reaches even higher. Keeping his hind legs and paws strong allows Bennie to arch slightly at the top of the pose. Breathing deeply, Bennie holds his backbend while gazing upward, before releasing downward on an exhale.

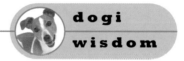
dogi wisdom

"Even on a rainy day, I salute the sun—I try to feel its energy above me and within me." —Bennie

chin, chest, knees

THE NEXT STAGE IN THE DOGA SUN SALUTATION IS CHIN, CHEST, KNEES, OR **ASHTANG PRANAM** (AHSH-TONG prah-NAHM). AFTER GREETING THE SUN ABOVE, THE DOGI BENDS TO GIVE RESPECT TO THE EARTH BELOW. IN THIS ASANA, THE CHEST, THE HOME OF THE HEART, KISSES THE EARTH.

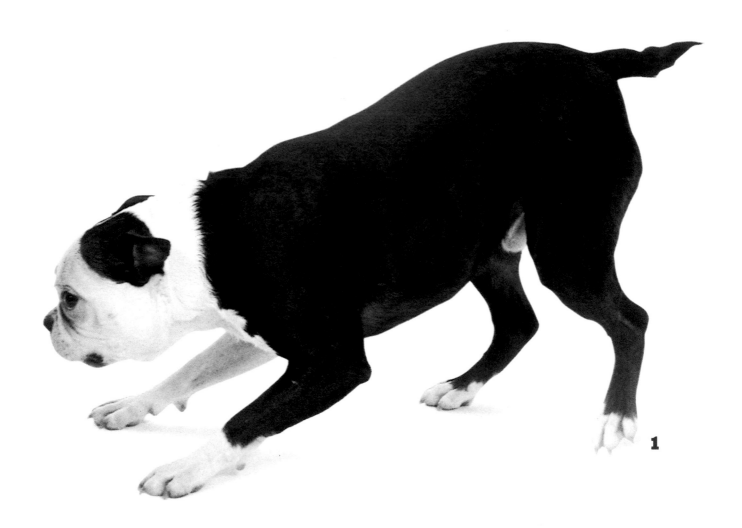

1

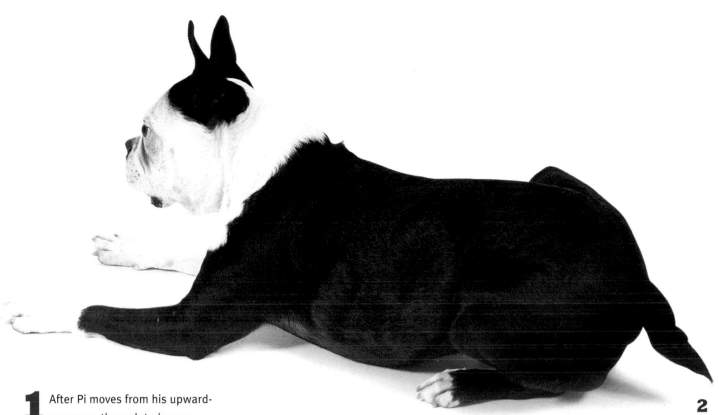

1 After Pi moves from his upward-paw pose through tadasana, he begins to lower himself down, chest first, toward the earth. Dogis not yet strong and flexible enough to actually touch the ground should think of blowing a kiss to the earth.

2 A different approach to chin, chest, knees is the sphinx variation. Pi lowers his entire front body downward all at once, and places his belly fully on the ground. This takes any strain off of his front legs. The feeling of reverence in the heart of the dogi is the key element to this part of the Sun Salutation.

2

human tip

Humans do this asana in reverse, as "knees, chest, chin," due to their different physical structure.

chaturanga

This pose, also known as the "doga push-up," can replace chin, chest, knees. It requires equal strength in all four legs to hold this pose.

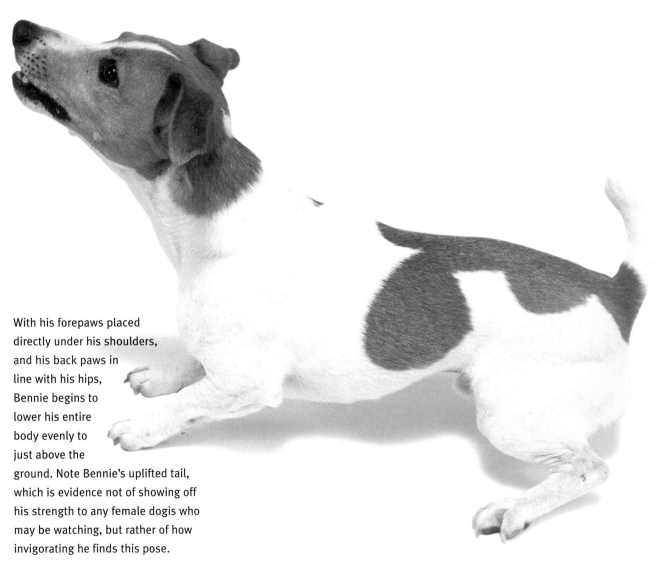

With his forepaws placed directly under his shoulders, and his back paws in line with his hips, Bennie begins to lower his entire body evenly to just above the ground. Note Bennie's uplifted tail, which is evidence not of showing off his strength to any female dogis who may be watching, but rather of how invigorating he finds this pose.

jump

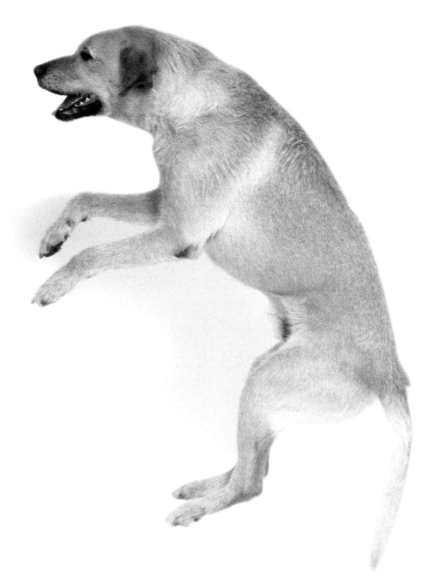

A MORE ADVANCED VARIATION
OF SUN SALUTATION INCLUDES
JUMPS FORWARD AND BACKWARD.
HOWEVER, IN DOGA, JUMPING
CAN ALSO BE DONE ON ITS OWN.

Each dogi has his own special reason
for jumping. Some are inspired by
treats held tantalizingly out of reach,
others by an urge to leap the back-
yard fence and chase skateboarders.
Buster is a dogi for whom jumping
is an expression of lightheartedness.
From a firmly grounded tadasana,
Buster bends, pressing his paws into
the ground. Drawing on the energy
he takes from the earth, Buster
springs upward.

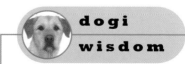

dogi wisdom

"Catching a ball is doga." —Buster

chair pose

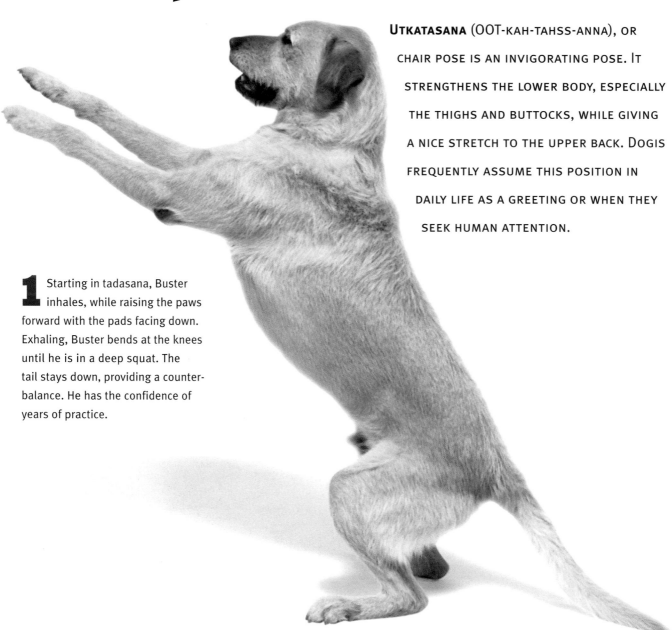

UTKATASANA (OOT-KAH-TAHSS-ANNA), OR CHAIR POSE IS AN INVIGORATING POSE. IT STRENGTHENS THE LOWER BODY, ESPECIALLY THE THIGHS AND BUTTOCKS, WHILE GIVING A NICE STRETCH TO THE UPPER BACK. DOGIS FREQUENTLY ASSUME THIS POSITION IN DAILY LIFE AS A GREETING OR WHEN THEY SEEK HUMAN ATTENTION.

1 Starting in tadasana, Buster inhales, while raising the paws forward with the pads facing down. Exhaling, Buster bends at the knees until he is in a deep squat. The tail stays down, providing a counter-balance. He has the confidence of years of practice.

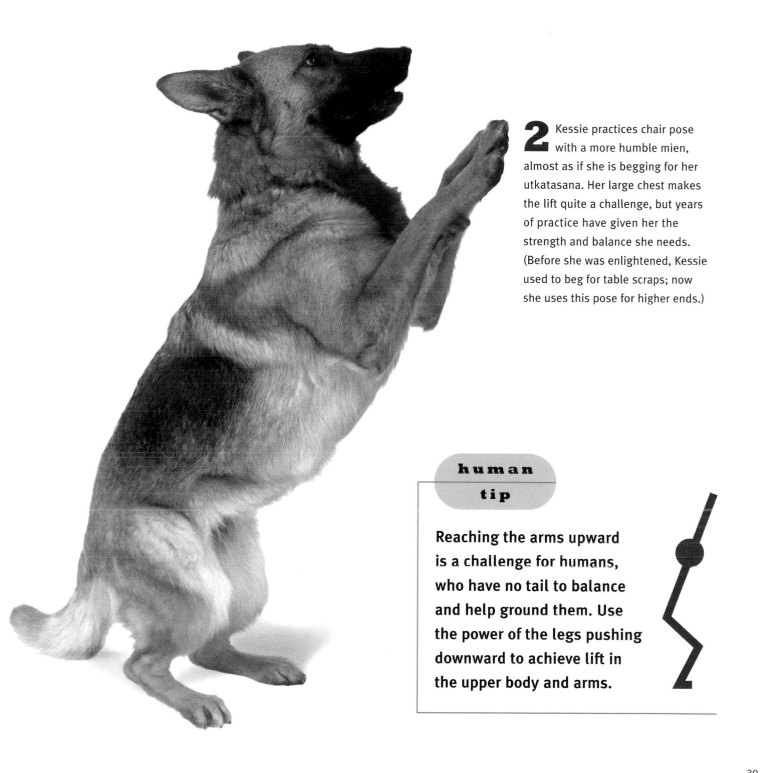

2 Kessie practices chair pose with a more humble mien, almost as if she is begging for her utkatasana. Her large chest makes the lift quite a challenge, but years of practice have given her the strength and balance she needs. (Before she was enlightened, Kessie used to beg for table scraps; now she uses this pose for higher ends.)

human tip

Reaching the arms upward is a challenge for humans, who have no tail to balance and help ground them. Use the power of the legs pushing downward to achieve lift in the upper body and arms.

warrior

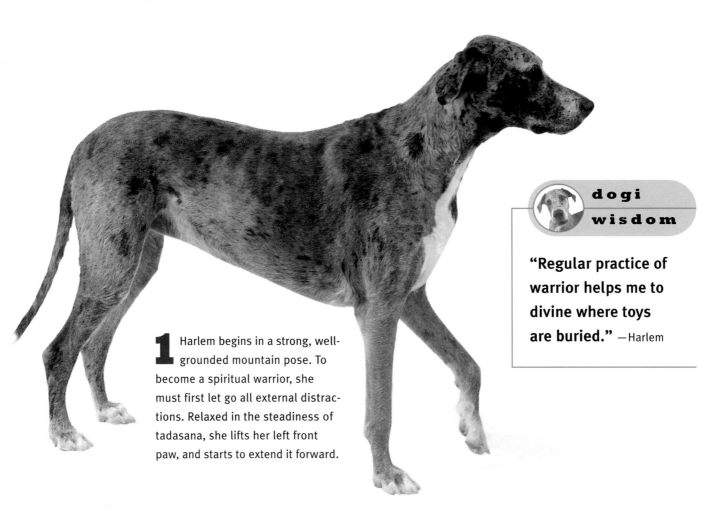

dogi wisdom

"Regular practice of warrior helps me to divine where toys are buried." —Harlem

1 Harlem begins in a strong, well-grounded mountain pose. To become a spiritual warrior, she must first let go all external distractions. Relaxed in the steadiness of tadasana, she lifts her left front paw, and starts to extend it forward.

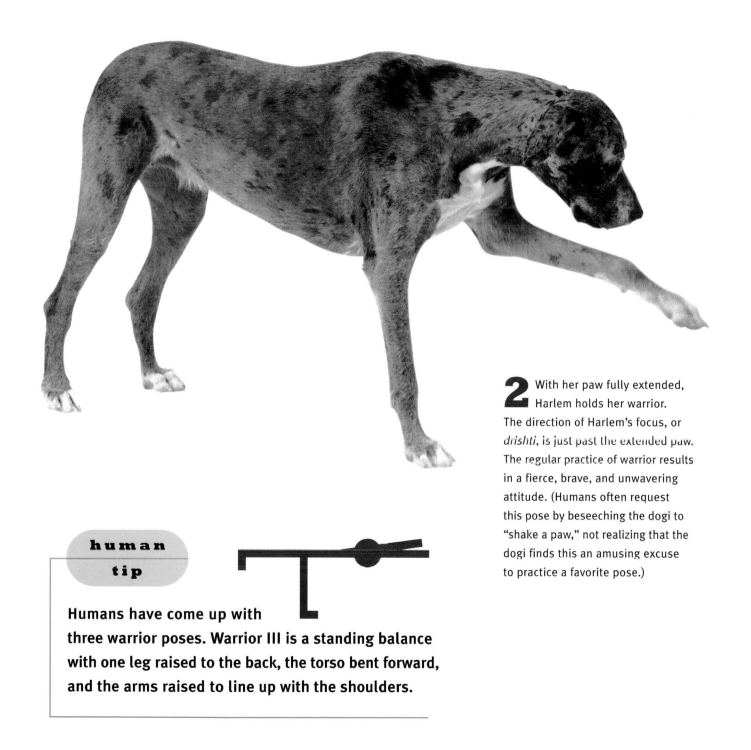

2 With her paw fully extended, Harlem holds her warrior. The direction of Harlem's focus, or *drishti*, is just past the extended paw. The regular practice of warrior results in a fierce, brave, and unwavering attitude. (Humans often request this pose by beseeching the dogi to "shake a paw," not realizing that the dogi finds this an amusing excuse to practice a favorite pose.)

human tip

Humans have come up with three warrior poses. Warrior III is a standing balance with one leg raised to the back, the torso bent forward, and the arms raised to line up with the shoulders.

triangle pose

Triangle pose, or **UTTHITA TRIKONASANA** (oo-TEE-tah trik-oh-NASS-anna), is a joyful, open, and embracing pose. Dogis do it with three paws on the ground and one lifted; the raised paw may be front or rear.

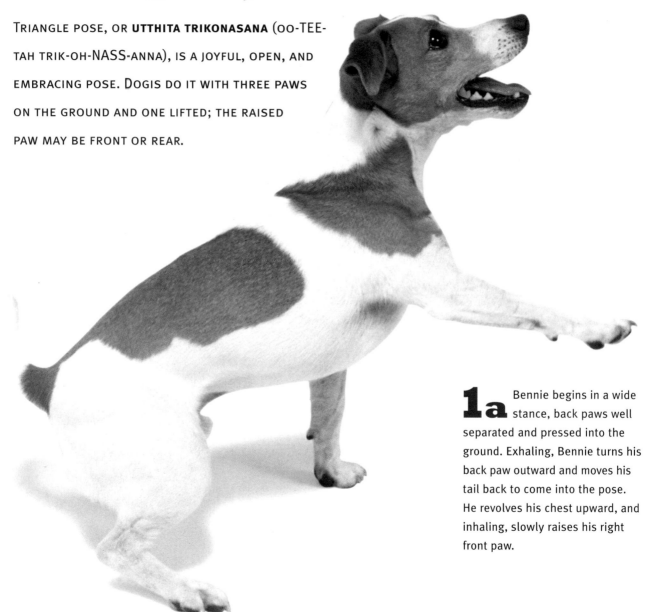

1a Bennie begins in a wide stance, back paws well separated and pressed into the ground. Exhaling, Bennie turns his back paw outward and moves his tail back to come into the pose. He revolves his chest upward, and inhaling, slowly raises his right front paw.

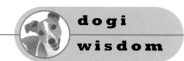

dogi wisdom

"During walks, I do triangle pose with my back leg lifted. I may do up to 20 repetitions during a walk around the block."

—Bennie

1b Deepening the pose, Bennie opens his chest to its fullest extent, then raises his paw even higher, achieving a tremendous stretch. Bennie does all of this with a rare simplicity. He seems to raise his paw and wave at the infinite.

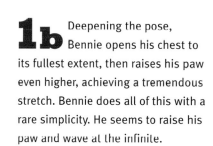

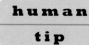

human tip

Yogis have adapted triangle for their bipedal stance. Bending from the hip, not the waist, lengthen both sides of the torso equally while extending the arms.

pup's pose

Dogis are careful to rest when poses become too intense. Pup's pose, or **BALASANA** (BAL-AHSS-anna) is the perfect resting place, and can be done before, during, or after practice. From this pose a dogi can choose to continue the practice or rest for the remainder of the afternoon.

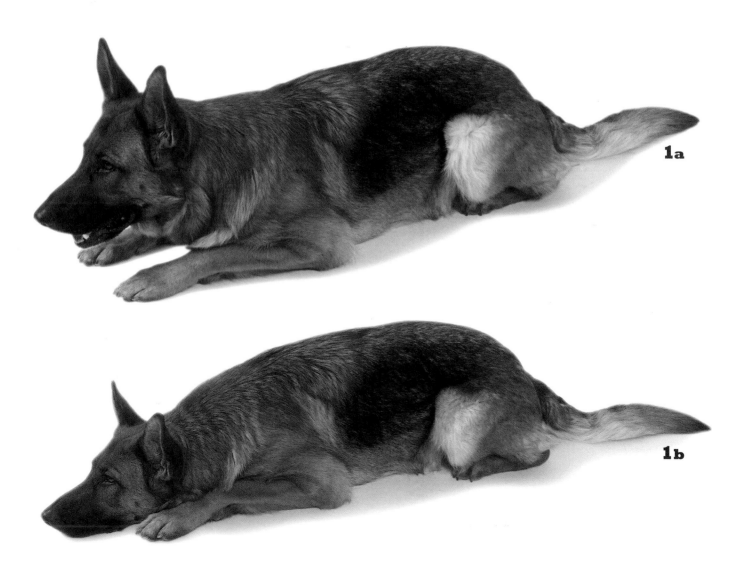

1a

1b

1a Typically a dogi will come into pup's pose from another pose such as downward-facing dog or upward-facing dog. Kessie moves into pup's pose by lowering her haunches and sitting back on her hind legs, tucking them comfortably and neatly underneath her. She then rests her elbows on the floor.

1b As she settles into the pose, Kessie checks for any remaining details in or around her that would hinder her relaxation. Then she extends her chin forward and rests it on the floor.

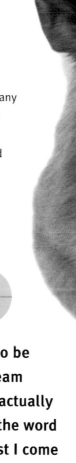

dogi wisdom

"Though I may seem to be lost in a doggy daydream during balasana, I am actually deeply alert. Mention the word 'walk,' and see how fast I come into tadasana." —Kessie

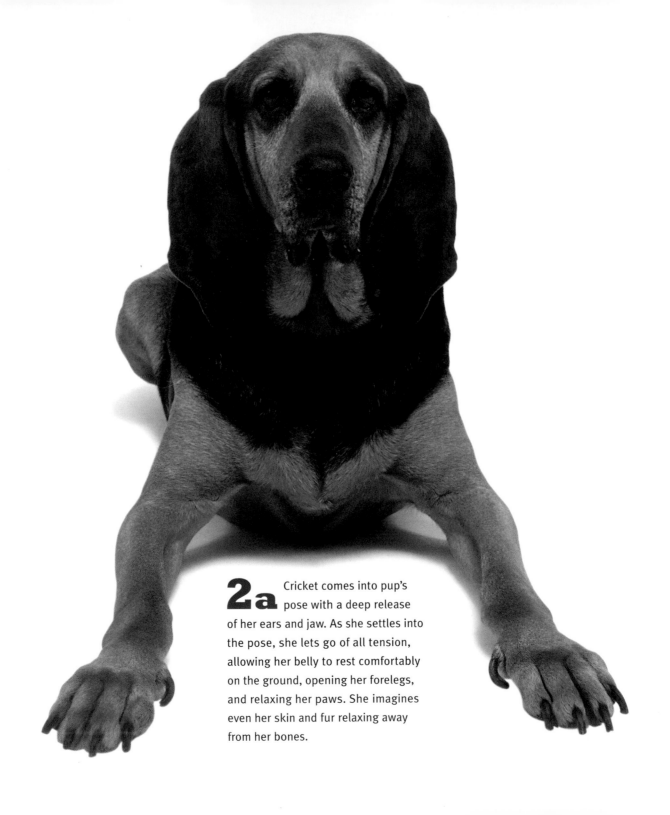

2a Cricket comes into pup's pose with a deep release of her ears and jaw. As she settles into the pose, she lets go of all tension, allowing her belly to rest comfortably on the ground, opening her forelegs, and relaxing her paws. She imagines even her skin and fur relaxing away from her bones.

2b Slowly sinking down into a full pup's pose, Cricket exhales fully, the breath fluttering her jowls as she lowers them to the floor. Her ears surrender to the relaxation.

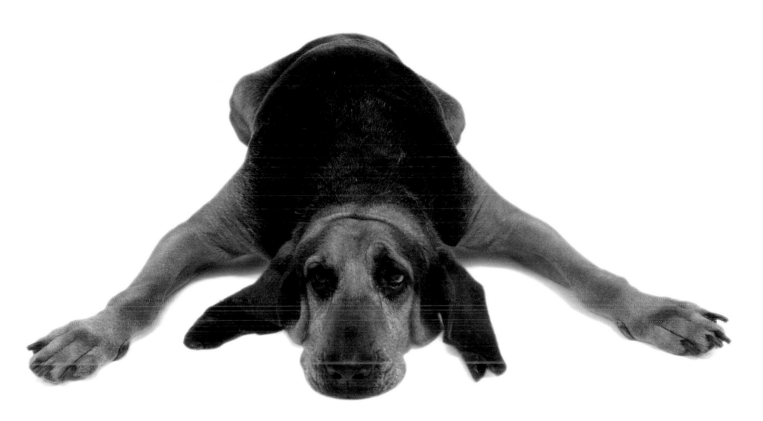

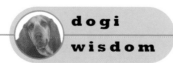 **dogi wisdom**

"For full enjoyment of balasana, try to relax your jowls fully into the ground." —Cricket

boat pose

PARIPURNA NAVASANA (PAR-EE-POOR-nah nah-VAHSS-anna), OR FULL BOAT POSE, IS A CHALLENGE TO THE DOGI'S ABDOMINAL STRENGTH AND SPINE FLEXIBILITY. MANY DOGIS APPRECIATE A BELLY RUB WHEN IN THIS POSE.

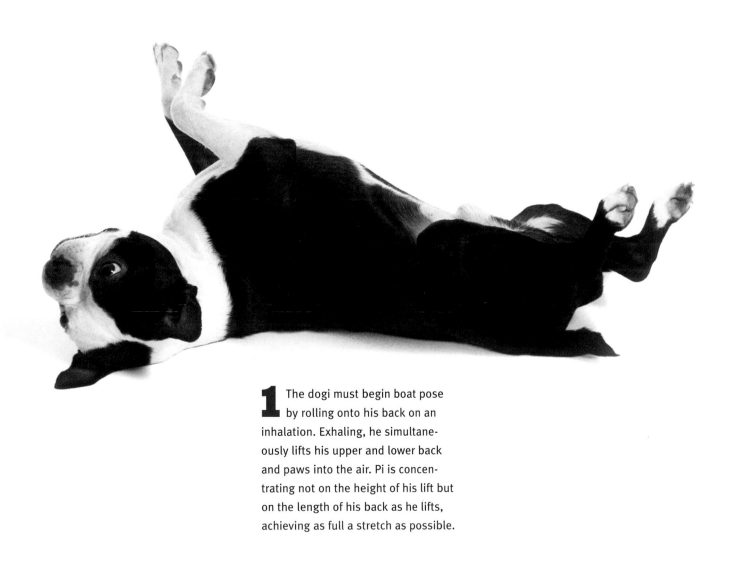

1 The dogi must begin boat pose by rolling onto his back on an inhalation. Exhaling, he simultaneously lifts his upper and lower back and paws into the air. Pi is concentrating not on the height of his lift but on the length of his back as he lifts, achieving as full a stretch as possible.

2 Like many dogis, Bennie does not lift very high into boat, but as he wriggles to lift up, his back and his abdomen gain strength. Humans should not mistake this wriggling for back-scratching.

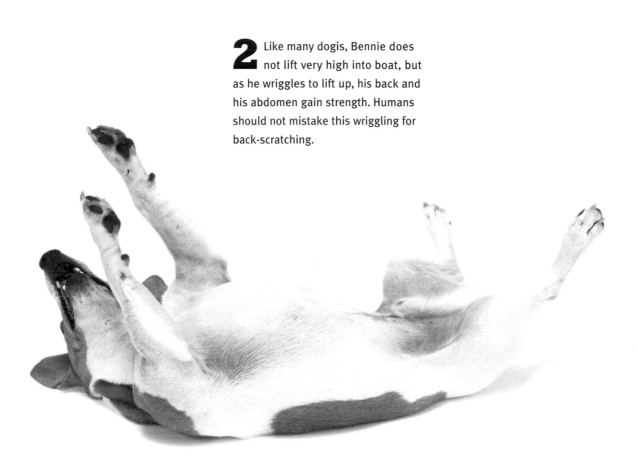

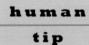

human tip

Humans have adapted this pose to balance on their buttocks. The real lesson of boat is perseverance when faced with a challenge.

cobra

Cobra pose, or **BHUJANGASANA** (boo-jahng-GAHSS-anna), is a position that appears in virtually every style of hatha doga. *Bhujanga* translates as "snake," and it is from these serpentine creatures that the first dogis adapted this belly-down posture. Cobra pose opens the chest and builds lower-back strength while invigorating the kidneys and nervous system. After performing this pose, many dogis will want to go for a walk.

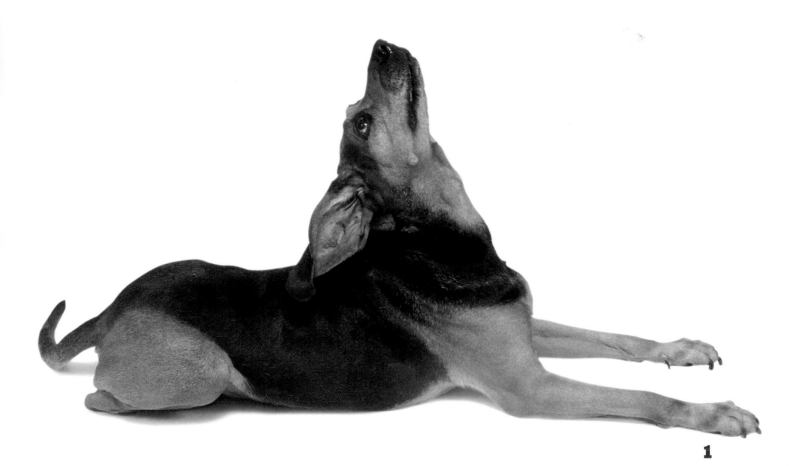

1

1 Cricket begins by lying on her belly, chin on the floor, front paws extended out in front of her, back legs curled beneath her. Pressing into her front legs and engaging the muscles in her upper back, Cricket inhales while lifting her head and upper chest off the floor. Now she resembles a serpent about to strike.

2 Keeping her shoulders down, Cricket inhales while lifting her head higher. She directs her gaze upward and back, and her ears fully open as she listens for inner wisdom.

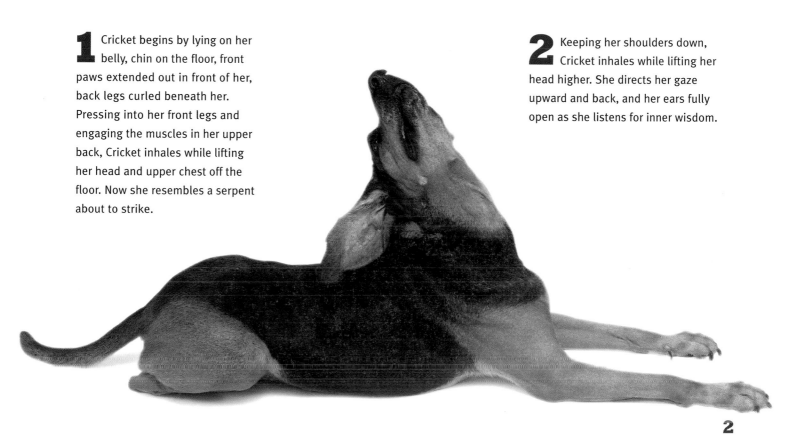

2

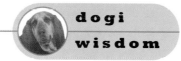

dogi wisdom

"Cobra enhances the dogi's sense of smell. Try practicing this pose while your human is cooking dinner." —Cricket

Without four paws to ground them, human yogis must focus instead on pressing the tops of their feet, thighs, and pelvis into the floor.

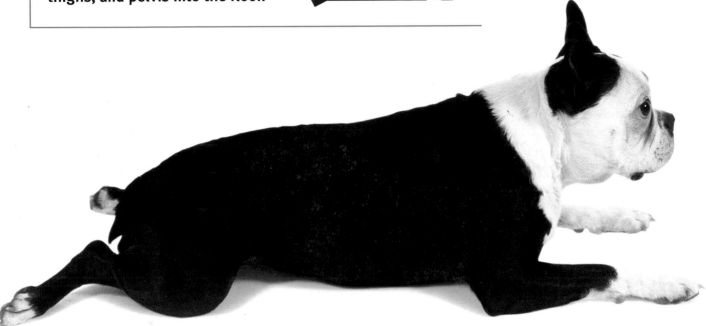

3 Pi's cobra is an excellent example of how an advanced dogi focuses on lengthening the spine before moving into a backward extension. By extending his neck forward, he creates space between each of his vertebra before arching his spine. This ability to focus on and try to perfect each aspect of the pose reveals the dogi's deep knowledge and understanding.

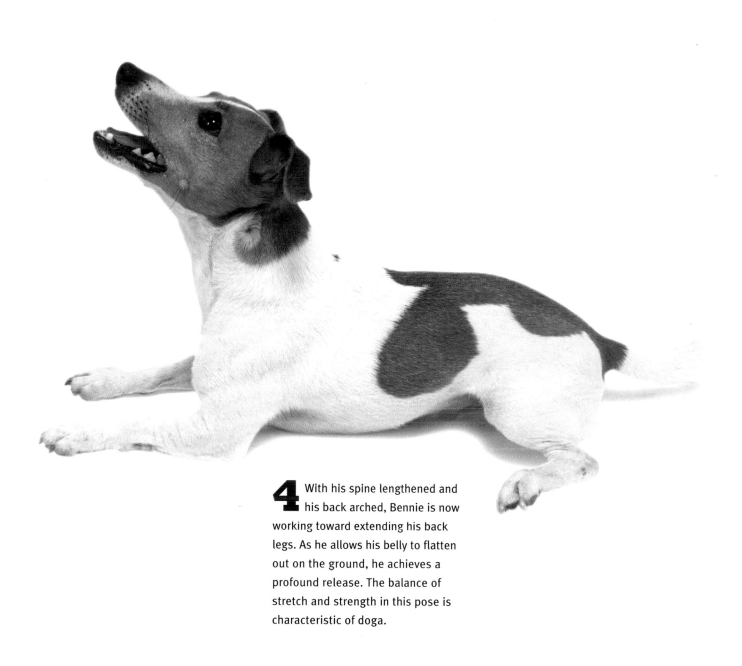

4 With his spine lengthened and his back arched, Bennie is now working toward extending his back legs. As he allows his belly to flatten out on the ground, he achieves a profound release. The balance of stretch and strength in this pose is characteristic of doga.

5 Harlem elongates from the very tip of her tail right to the crown of her head. She keeps her throat soft, enabling her to lengthen at the base of her skull, lifting her head away from her shoulders. She is not in a hurry to arch her back.

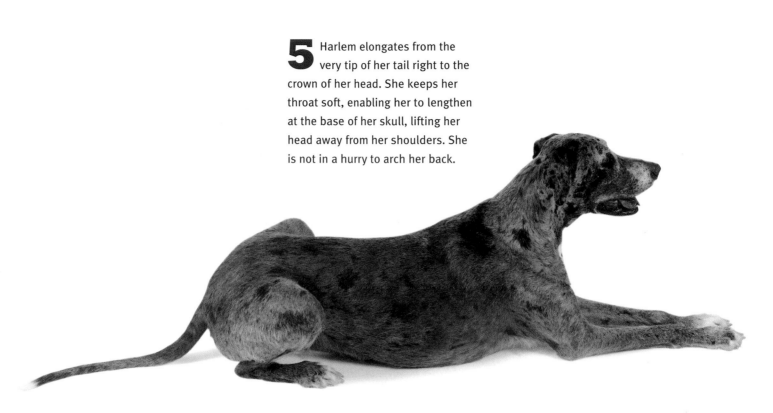

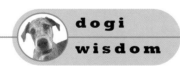 **dogi wisdom**

"Cobra both opens the heart and stimulates digestion. I practice it before and after dinner." —Harlem

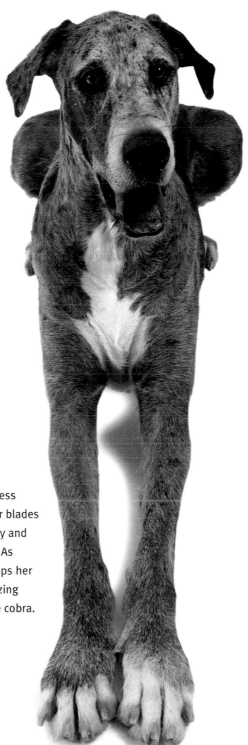

6 Harlem's front legs press down and her shoulder blades are firm. This creates stability and elegance in her upper body. As she raises her head, she drops her ears down and back, visualizing that they are the hood of the cobra.

seated twist

TWISTS ARE AN IMPORTANT PART OF DOGA; THEY MASSAGE THE INTERNAL ORGANS WHILE ENHANCING FLEXIBILITY AND RELEASING TENSION. THE SEATED TWIST, OR **ARDHA MATSEYENDRASANA** (AR-DUH MOTT-SAY-EN-DRAHSS-ANNA) ENCOURAGES LENGTHENING IN THE SPINE, OPENING OF THE SHOULDERS, AND MOBILITY IN THE NECK, WHILE ALSO ALLOWING THE DOGI TO LOOK AROUND WITHOUT GETTING UP.

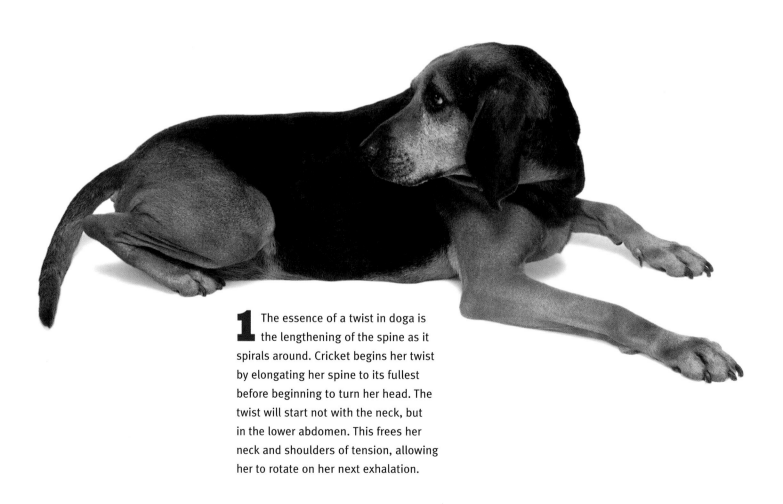

1 The essence of a twist in doga is the lengthening of the spine as it spirals around. Cricket begins her twist by elongating her spine to its fullest before beginning to turn her head. The twist will start not with the neck, but in the lower abdomen. This frees her neck and shoulders of tension, allowing her to rotate on her next exhalation.

2a Hip position is critical in a doga twist. Note how Cricket's hips are aligned forward. She is also careful to ground herself, pressing into the floor with her tucked-under back legs.

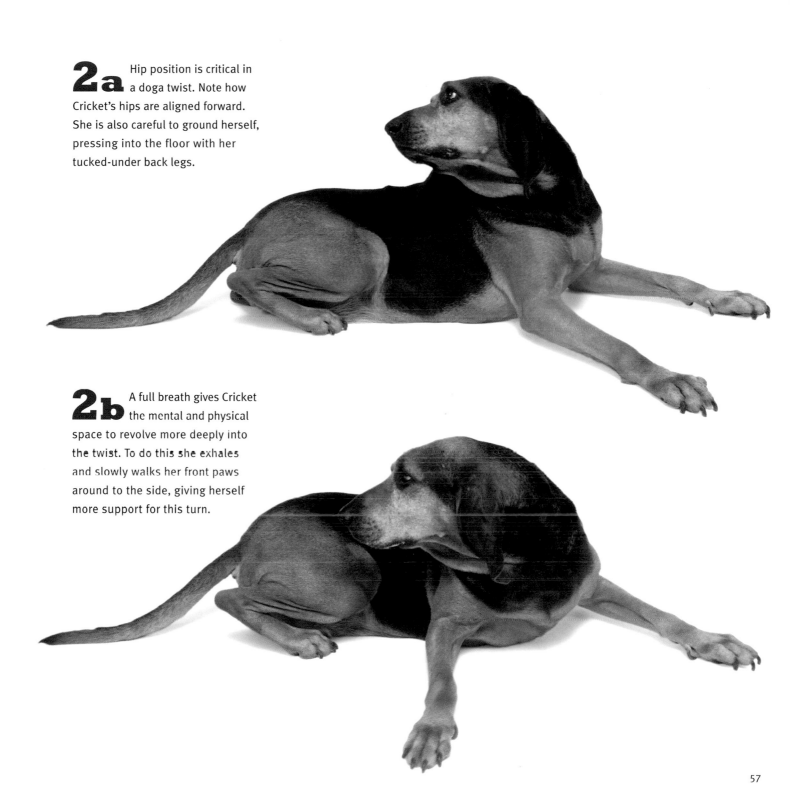

2b A full breath gives Cricket the mental and physical space to revolve more deeply into the twist. To do this she exhales and slowly walks her front paws around to the side, giving herself more support for this turn.

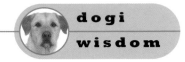
"When I have a stressful day, I find seated twist relieves my tension." —Buster

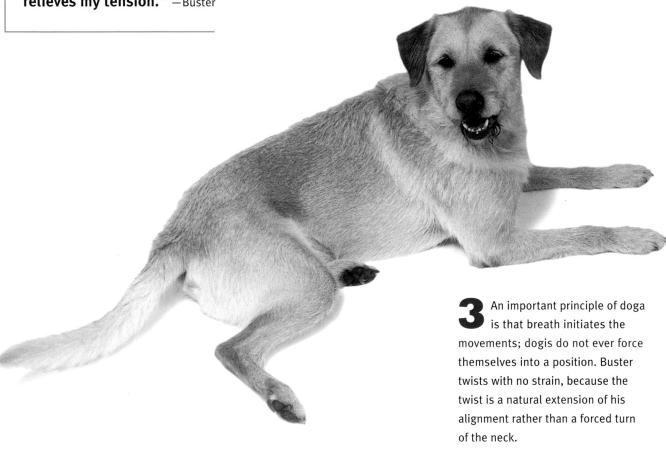

3 An important principle of doga is that breath initiates the movements; dogis do not ever force themselves into a position. Buster twists with no strain, because the twist is a natural extension of his alignment rather than a forced turn of the neck.

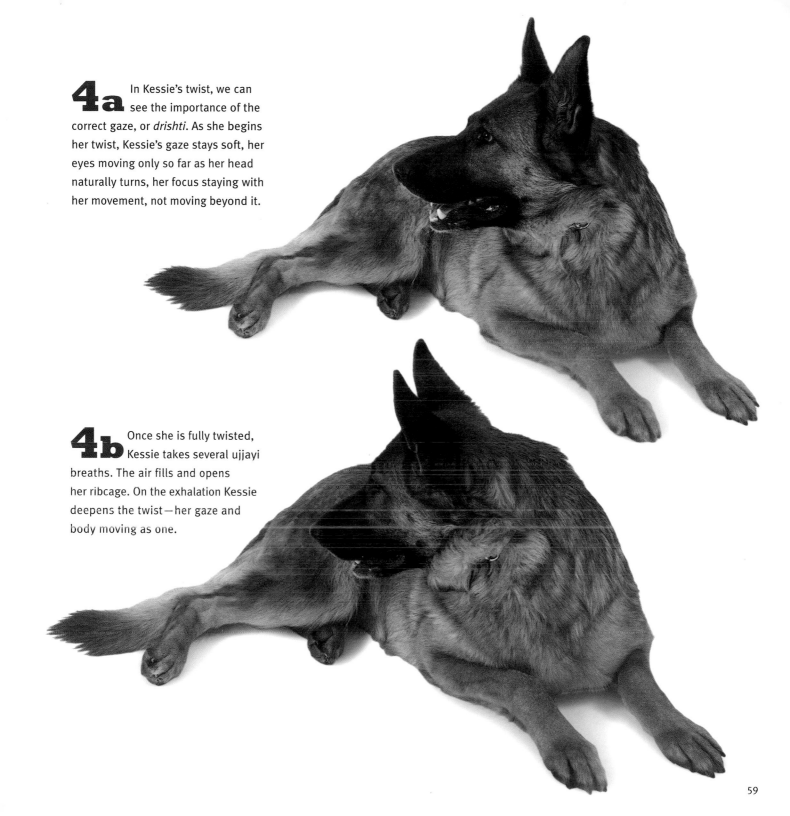

4a In Kessie's twist, we can see the importance of the correct gaze, or *drishti*. As she begins her twist, Kessie's gaze stays soft, her eyes moving only so far as her head naturally turns, her focus staying with her movement, not moving beyond it.

4b Once she is fully twisted, Kessie takes several ujjayi breaths. The air fills and opens her ribcage. On the exhalation Kessie deepens the twist—her gaze and body moving as one.

lion pose

THE SANSKRIT WORD *SIMHA* MEANS "POWERFUL ONE" AND IS ALSO THE WORD FOR "LION." THUS, A DOGI PERFORMING **SIMHASANA** (SIM-HASS-ANNA), OR LION POSE, RESEMBLES A ROARING LION, BOTH OUTWARDLY AND INWARDLY, AS HE EXPERIENCES HIS OWN LIONLIKE QUALITIES OF COURAGE, VIRTUE, AND NOBILITY. IT ALSO RELIEVES TENSION IN THE JAW, PREVENTS SORE THROATS, SMOOTHES A ROUGH BARK, AND SWEETENS DOGI BREATH.

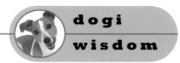

dogi wisdom

"In this pose I repeat to myself: 'I will protect my home from mailmen, raccoons, and other threats.'" —Bennie

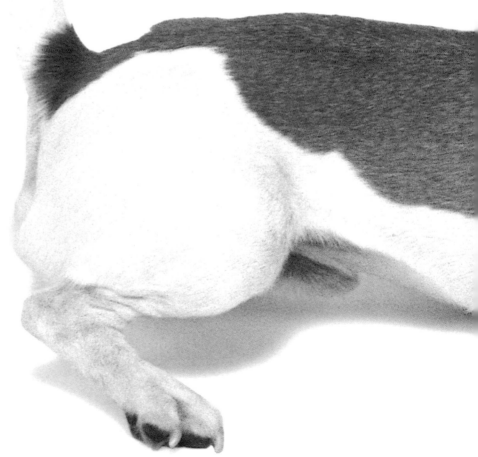

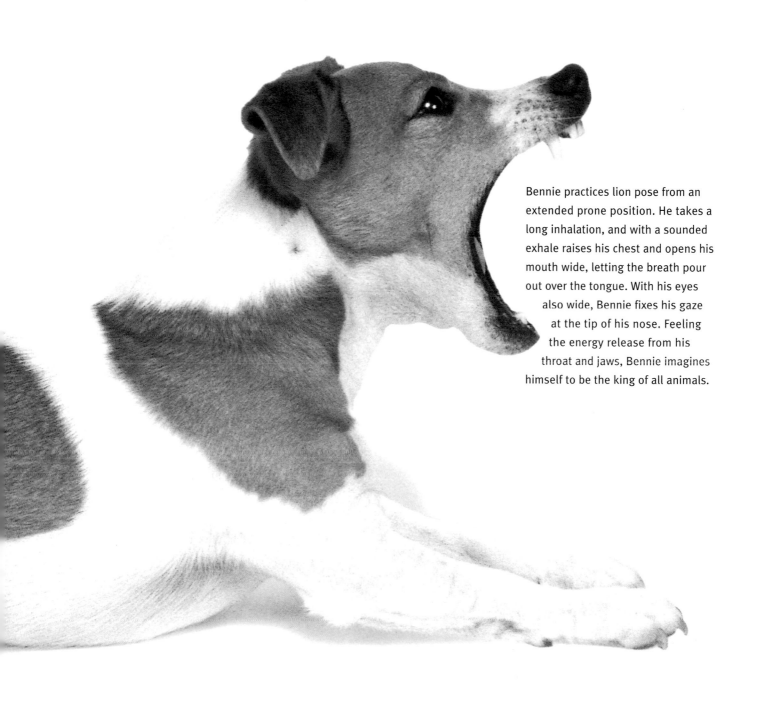

Bennie practices lion pose from an extended prone position. He takes a long inhalation, and with a sounded exhale raises his chest and opens his mouth wide, letting the breath pour out over the tongue. With his eyes also wide, Bennie fixes his gaze at the tip of his nose. Feeling the energy release from his throat and jaws, Bennie imagines himself to be the king of all animals.

happy puppy

A FAVORITE POSE OF DOGIS AT EVERY LEVEL, **HAPPY PUPPY** IS A TRUE EXPRESSION OF THE SHEER JOY OF DOGA. HAPPY PUPPY POSE IS A VARIATION ON A CLASSICAL ASANA SERIES CALLED **SUPTA PADANGUSTHASANA** (SOUP-TAH POD-ANG-GOOSH-TAHSS-ANNA) THAT CAN BE RESTORATIVE AND COOLING. HAPPY PUPPY IS ALSO A POSE THAT BOTH PUPPIES AND HUMAN BABIES DO SO NATURALLY THAT "LEARNING" IT SEEMS UNNECESSARY.

1 Bennie inhales while rolling onto his back, lifting all four legs into the air. He presses his spine down into the floor as he waves his paws at the ceiling. While keeping his shoulders and the back of his neck resting on the floor, Bennie exhales and relaxes his whole spine into the ground.

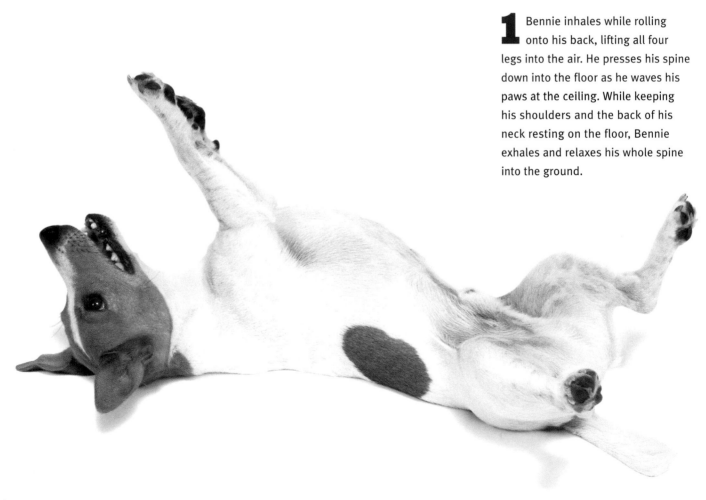

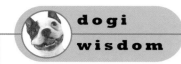
"My mantra for happy puppy: 'Rub my tummy, rub my tummy.' I repeat it throughout the pose." —Pi

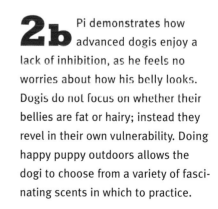

2a With his spine fully lengthened on the ground, Pi opens the front of his body fully, allowing his front legs to relax downward and his hind legs to settle into openness. He uses the smoothness of his breath to guide him.

2b Pi demonstrates how advanced dogis enjoy a lack of inhibition, as he feels no worries about how his belly looks. Dogis do not focus on whether their bellies are fat or hairy; instead they revel in their own vulnerability. Doing happy puppy outdoors allows the dogi to choose from a variety of fascinating scents in which to practice.

shake and roll

SHAKES AND ROLLS ARE USED BY DOGIS DURING TRANSITIONS FROM ONE POSE TO ANOTHER, ALLOWING THEM TO FULLY SHAKE OFF THE ESSENCE OF ONE ASANA BEFORE GIVING THEMSELVES TO THE NEXT. SHAKES AND ROLLS ARE AT ONCE RELAXING AND STIMULATING, PUTTING THE DOGI INTO THE PERFECT FRAME OF MIND FOR BEGINNING A NEW POSE.

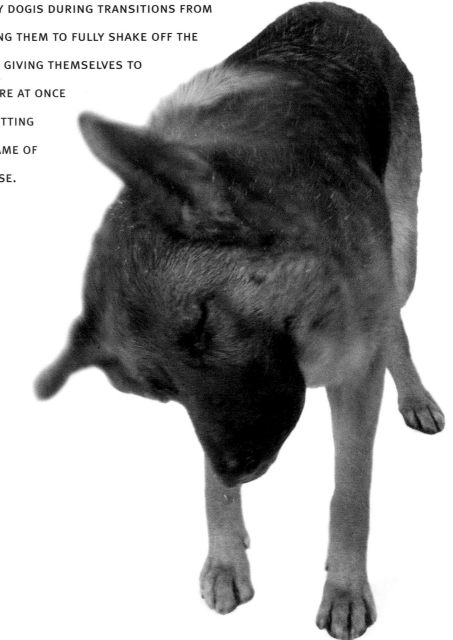

1 For Kessie, shaking out her body is like taking a big breath into and around each strand of fur. She begins in a firmly grounded tadasana, then on an exhale begins to shake her torso vigorously. A lot of wind is created when she does this, and she enjoys the feeling of her ears flapping in the breeze.

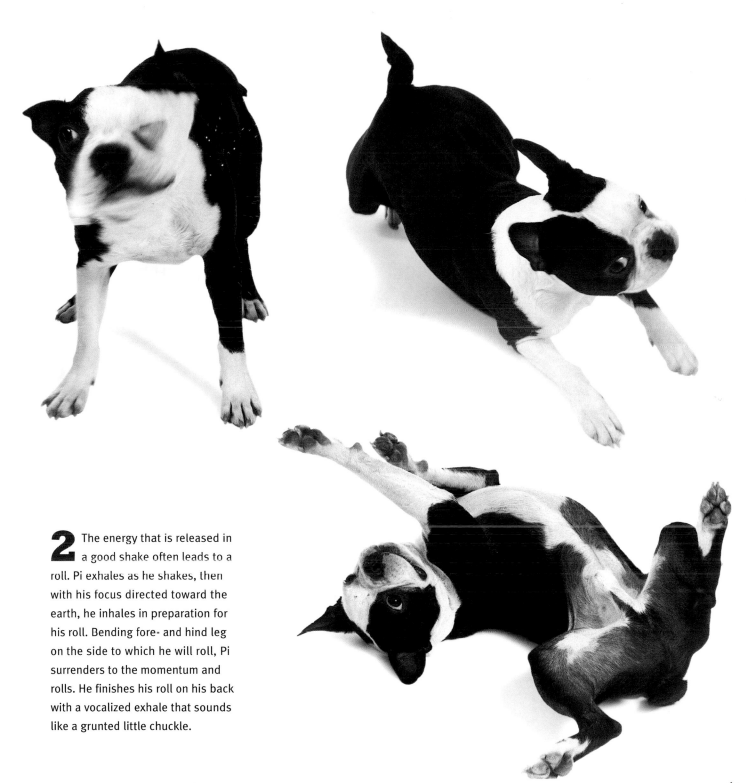

2 The energy that is released in a good shake often leads to a roll. Pi exhales as he shakes, then with his focus directed toward the earth, he inhales in preparation for his roll. Bending fore- and hind leg on the side to which he will roll, Pi surrenders to the momentum and rolls. He finishes his roll on his back with a vocalized exhale that sounds like a grunted little chuckle.

shoulder-opening poses

FREEDOM IN THE JOINTS IS AN IMPORTANT GOAL. OPENING THE SHOULDERS IS OF PARTICULAR VALUE TO THE DOGI (AND YOGI), AS IT IMPROVES POSTURE, OPENS THE CHEST, AND RELEASES TENSION—ALL OF WHICH ALLOW FOR BETTER, DEEPER BREATHING, WHICH LEADS TO A CLEAR, CALM MIND—THE ESSENCE OF THE PRACTICE.

dogi wisdom

"In shoulder-opening poses, I also open my heart, which brings love and attention, and occasionally treats, my way." —Harlem

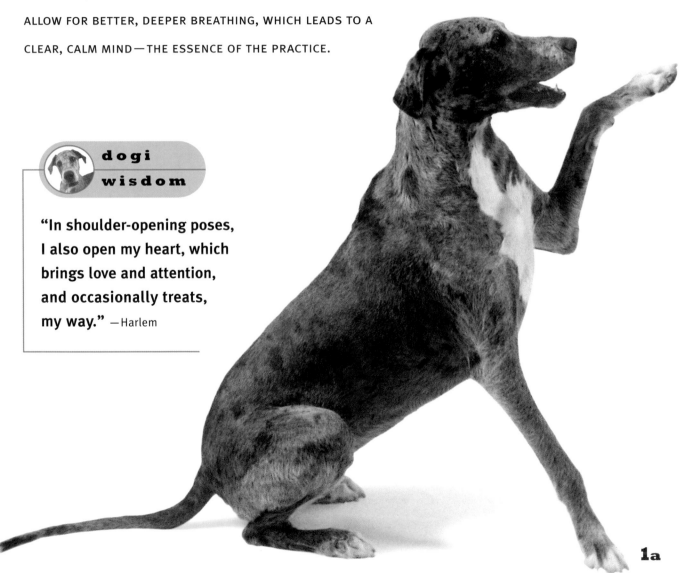

1a

1a Harlem demonstrates a typical doga shoulder-opening pose that humans may recognize as the "shake a paw" position, but dogis call shoulder opening with one raised paw. From her firmly seated posture, Harlem reaches her left front paw forward, feeling it become light.

1b As Harlem breathes, her chest and ribs expand more fully. Her opening evolves naturally with the lifting of her right paw, as she moves into shoulder opening with two raised paws. As the dogi works on opening her shoulders and lifting her chest, her connection to the ground below also deepens, and she feels the powerful energy of the earth moving through her.

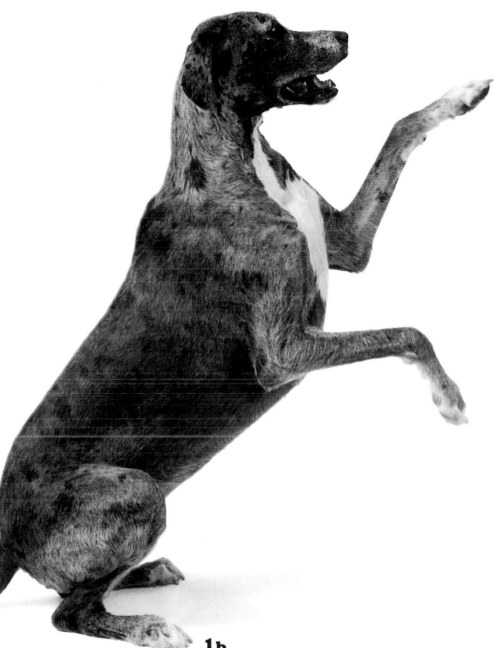

1b

hip-opening poses

The active dogi's daily regimen of walking, running, and jumping tends to shorten muscles and ligaments, and reduce flexibility. As a result, many doga poses are devoted to opening the hips.

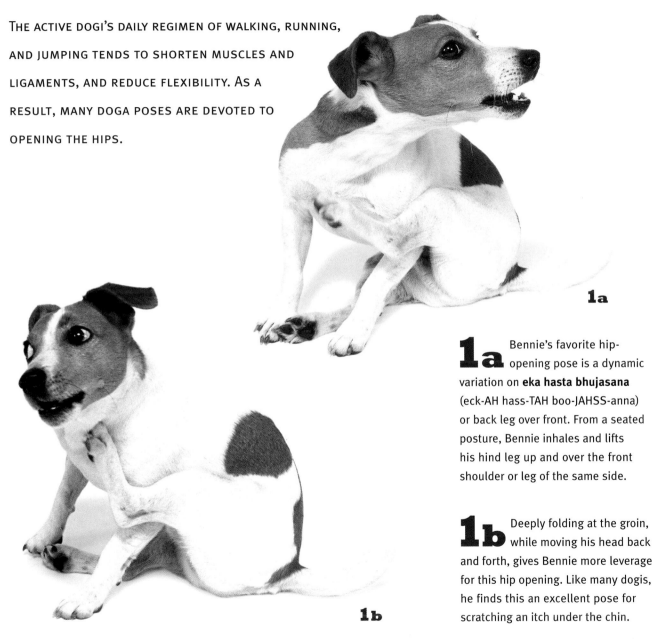

1a

1a Bennie's favorite hip-opening pose is a dynamic variation on **eka hasta bhujasana** (eck-AH hass-TAH boo-JAHSS-anna) or back leg over front. From a seated posture, Bennie inhales and lifts his hind leg up and over the front shoulder or leg of the same side.

1b Deeply folding at the groin, while moving his head back and forth, gives Bennie more leverage for this hip opening. Like many dogis, he finds this an excellent pose for scratching an itch under the chin.

1b

2a Pi's open hips are a result of long practice of this pose, a variation on frog, or **bhekasana** (buh-KAHSS-anna). From a seated pose, he releases into a forward prone position, spreads his hind legs, and releases his groin completely to the floor.

2b Because Pi is free from deeply rooted inhibitions, he is able to lay his belly and pelvis right down on the ground. He is deeply relaxed yet also quite alert.

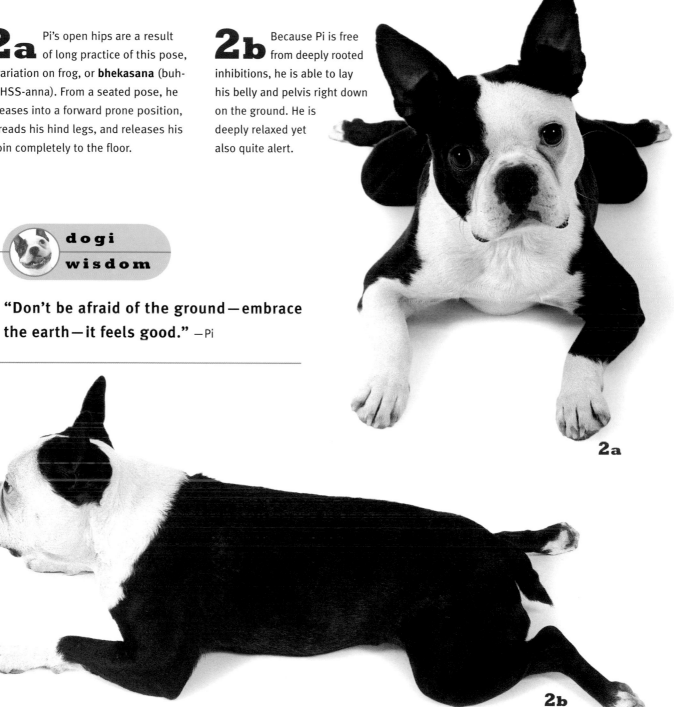

dogi wisdom

"Don't be afraid of the ground—embrace the earth—it feels good." —Pi

2a

2b

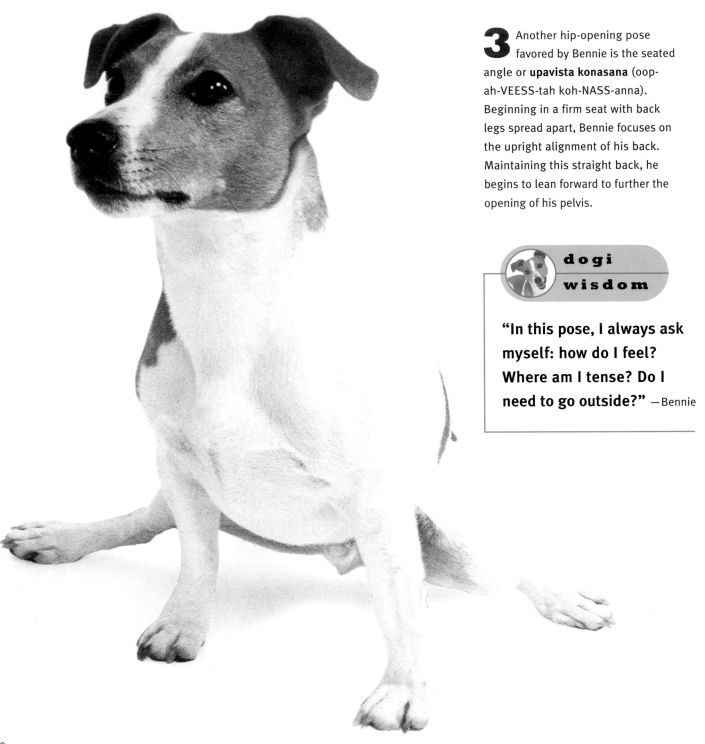

3 Another hip-opening pose favored by Bennie is the seated angle or **upavista konasana** (oop-ah-VEESS-tah koh-NASS-anna). Beginning in a firm seat with back legs spread apart, Bennie focuses on the upright alignment of his back. Maintaining this straight back, he begins to lean forward to further the opening of his pelvis.

dogi wisdom

"In this pose, I always ask myself: how do I feel? Where am I tense? Do I need to go outside?" —Bennie

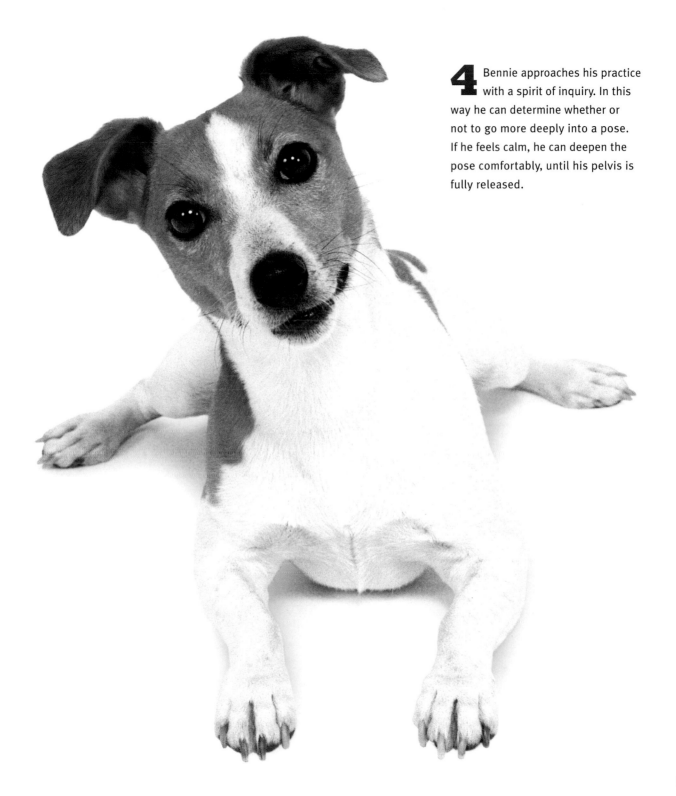

4 Bennie approaches his practice with a spirit of inquiry. In this way he can determine whether or not to go more deeply into a pose. If he feels calm, he can deepen the pose comfortably, until his pelvis is fully released.

lotus pose

ONE OF THE MOST WELL-KNOWN POSES IN DOGA IS THE LOTUS POSE, OR **PADMASANA** (POD-MAHSS-ANNA). WHEN SEATED IN THIS CROSS-LEGGED POSE, THE DOGI'S PAWS RESEMBLE THE PETALS OF A LOTUS FLOWER (IN SANSKRIT, *PADMA* MEANS "LOTUS"). REVERED AS A MEDITATION POSTURE, PADMASANA CALMS THE MIND AND ENHANCES CONCENTRATION. IT IS ALSO EXCELLENT FOR PRANAYAMA, OR BREATHING PRACTICE.

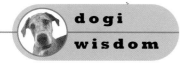

dogi wisdom

"In preparation for lotus, I like to turn in a circle three times before sitting down." —Harlem

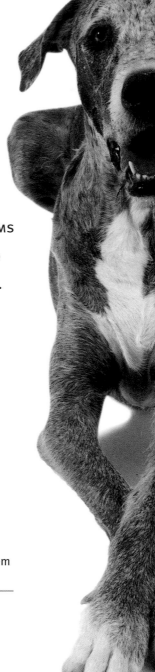

1

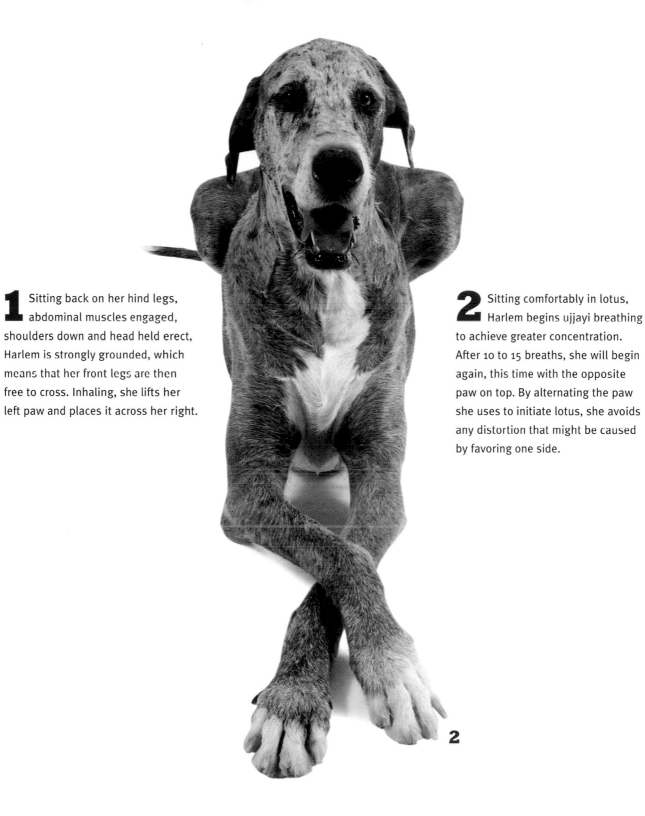

1 Sitting back on her hind legs, abdominal muscles engaged, shoulders down and head held erect, Harlem is strongly grounded, which means that her front legs are then free to cross. Inhaling, she lifts her left paw and places it across her right.

2 Sitting comfortably in lotus, Harlem begins ujjayi breathing to achieve greater concentration. After 10 to 15 breaths, she will begin again, this time with the opposite paw on top. By alternating the paw she uses to initiate lotus, she avoids any distortion that might be caused by favoring one side.

2

corpse pose

DOGA SESSIONS ALWAYS CONCLUDE WITH A PERIOD OF DEEP RELAXATION, IN WHICH THE DOGI RECLINES AND LETS GO OF ALL MENTAL AND PHYSICAL EFFORT. THIS IS THE CORPSE POSE, OR **SAVASANA** (SHA-VAHSS-ANNA). IN SAVASANA, THE DOGI'S BODY IS STILL AS HE OBSERVES HIS MIND. THIS IS NOT A TIME TO SLEEP, BUT RATHER TO BE TRANQUIL YET AWARE. DOGIS ARE HIGHLY GIFTED IN THE ART OF RELAXATION, AND HUMANS CAN LEARN MUCH FROM THEM IN THIS REGARD.

1 As Kessie prepares for savasana, she lies down on her side. She precisely aligns her right shoulder over her left shoulder and her right hip over her left hip, in a position that is natural and comfortable. She releases her jaw and covers her back legs with the warmth of her tail. She takes a few slow, deep breaths to facilitate her relaxation, then allows herself to breathe naturally, merely observing.

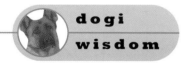

dogi wisdom

"Do not allow outward disturbances ('do I hear the mailman?') or private worries ('are we going to the vet today?') to distract you. Let it all go." —Kessie

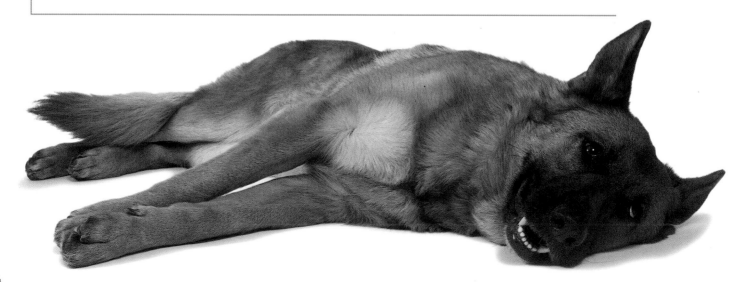

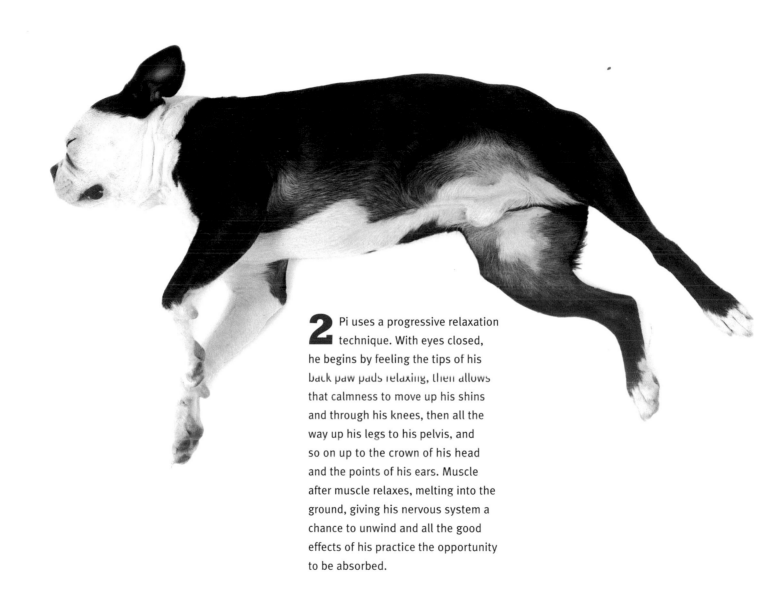

2 Pi uses a progressive relaxation technique. With eyes closed, he begins by feeling the tips of his back paw pads relaxing, then allows that calmness to move up his shins and through his knees, then all the way up his legs to his pelvis, and so on up to the crown of his head and the points of his ears. Muscle after muscle relaxes, melting into the ground, giving his nervous system a chance to unwind and all the good effects of his practice the opportunity to be absorbed.

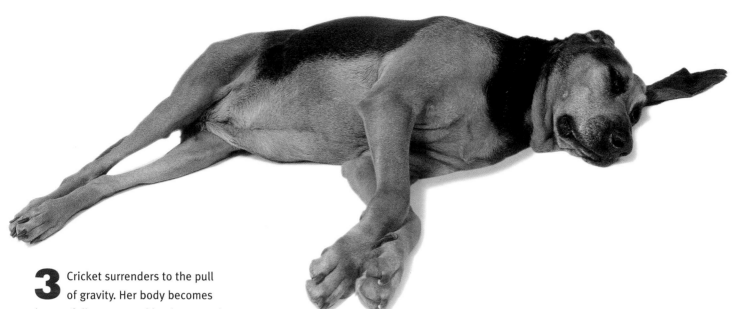

3 Cricket surrenders to the pull of gravity. Her body becomes heavy; fully supported by the ground, she can completely yield. Gently easing away any final vestiges of tension, she relaxes her tongue, her nostrils, and the channels of her ears. She releases her forehead and eyebrows, and lets her eyes slowly droop shut. Still and serene, she observes her breath. If her thoughts drift toward daily matters such as dinner, she quietly brings herself back into the moment with a few deep breaths, and refocuses inward.

human tip

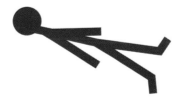

Dogic relaxation is so profound that many yogis study for years to be able to attain a similar state. Humans find it best to practice savasana while lying on the back, with the legs allowed to fall slightly open, and the arms at a slight angle to the body, palms open, eyes closed, breathing natural. In this pose, begin to feel relaxation spreading through body and mind; let go of tension.

4 After resting quietly in savasana for several minutes (or has it been hours?), Bennie is ready to get up. Dogis know that it is best to come out of savasana slowly, taking some time to reconnect with their surroundings. Bennie gently opens his eyes, refocusing his attention outward. He takes several deeper breaths, and begins to stretch his legs. His ears perk up, becoming attentive to the sounds around him, and his tail begins to lift. When he is ready, he will roll into a sitting position.

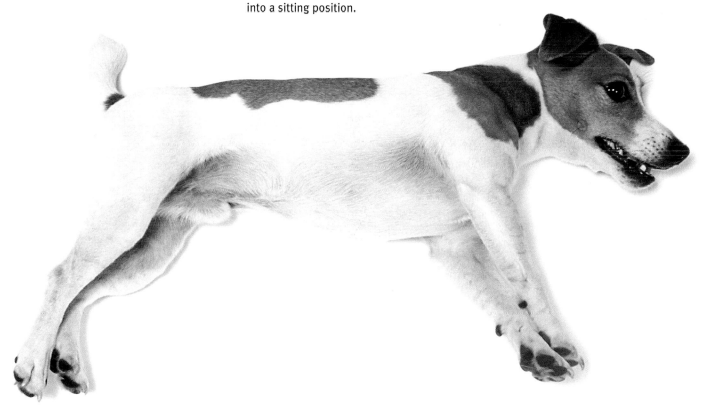

sense withdrawal

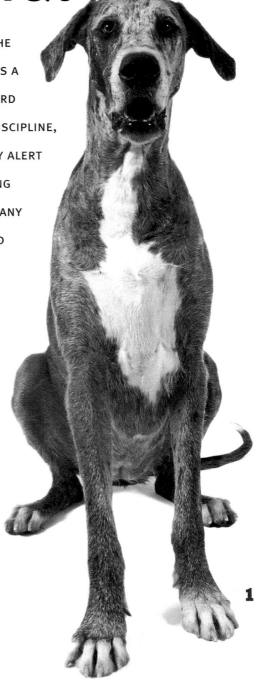

SENSE WITHDRAWAL, OR **PRATYAHARA** (PRUHT-YAH-HAH-RAH), IS THE PREREQUISITE TO MEDITATION. DURING THIS STAGE THE DOGI MAKES A CONSCIOUS EFFORT TO DRAW THE AWARENESS OF HIS SENSES INWARD AND DETACH FROM OUTSIDE STIMULATION. THIS REQUIRES GREAT DISCIPLINE, AS A DOGI'S EYES, EARS, NOSE, TONGUE, AND SKIN ARE CONSTANTLY ALERT TO NEW SENSATIONS. SENSE WITHDRAWAL HELPS THE DOGI TO BRING THE OBJECTS OF HIS DESIRES (TREATS, RANK SMELLS, OR THE COMPANY OF OTHER DOGIS) UNDER CONTROL. AT LAST, THE DOGI IS LIBERATED FROM HIS OWN CRAVINGS.

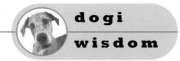

dogi wisdom

"Until my human learned to recognize pratyahara, she thought I was stubbornly refusing to come when called. Now she sees that my senses are inwardly directed." —Harlem

1

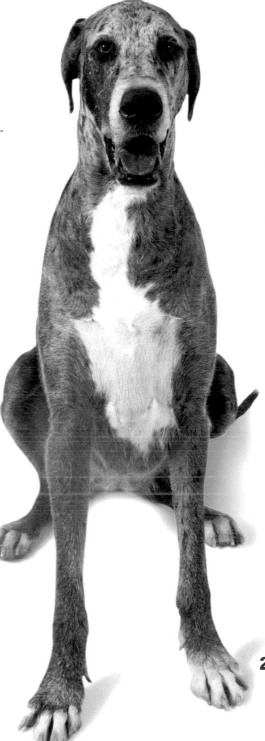

1 Harlem prepares for sense withdrawal. She sits in an easy but stable posture, rump and hind paws firmly settled, forepaws planted, head up, ears lifted and open. She is aware of her breath, observing but not controlling it, aware of but not engaged with the outside world.

2 After several minutes of following her breath, Harlem is ready to begin sense withdrawal. She slowly draws her ear flaps down and closes them over her ear openings. Then she visualizes the trail of her ear canals, consciously opening, softening, and deepening the inner ears. During this process, Harlem experiences a profound relaxation as the external world fades from her consciousness.

2

meditation

UNLIKE HUMANS, DOGIS DO NOT REQUIRE FORMAL INSTRUCTION IN MEDITATION, OR **DHAYANA** (DYAH-nah).

DOGIS ARE NATURAL MEDITATORS, CONTINUALLY IN A STATE OF AWARENESS, TOTALLY PRESENT IN EACH

MOMENT, AND WILLING TO LET GO. NEVERTHELESS, MANY DOGIS FOLLOW TECHNIQUES THAT HELP THEM

ACHIEVE THE MEDITATIVE STATE: CALM, QUIET IN THE MIND, AWARE OF EVERYTHING AT ONCE, YET NOTHING

IN PARTICULAR. IT IS A STATE OF NON-JUDGMENT AND INACTION.

THE DOGI SIMPLY IS.

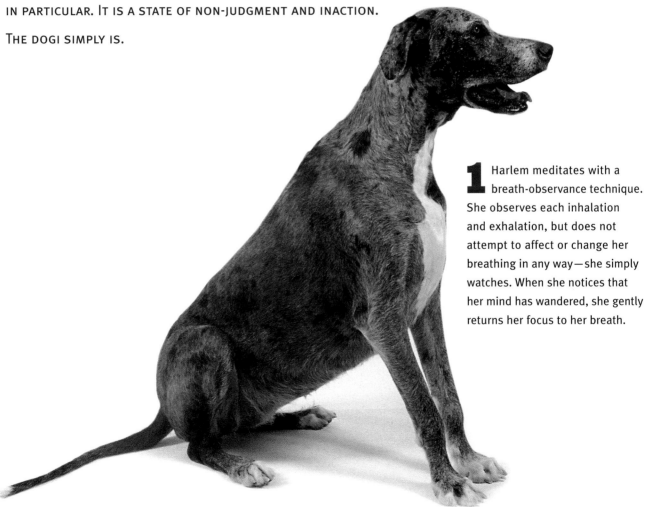

1 Harlem meditates with a breath-observance technique. She observes each inhalation and exhalation, but does not attempt to affect or change her breathing in any way—she simply watches. When she notices that her mind has wandered, she gently returns her focus to her breath.

2 Pi prepares himself for loving-kindness meditation by taking a few slow, deep breaths. Returning to his normal breath, he begins to silently repeat the phrases, "May I be happy. May I be healthy. May I be safe. May I live with peace." Feeling each word, he repeats the phrases to himself in a rhythm that feels comfortable. He then directs these wishes to different beings: first his human companion whom he loves, then a dogi down the block for whom he has neutral feelings, and finally a squirrel whom he hates from the bottom of his scruff. "May you be happy. May you be healthy. May you..."

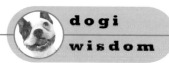

dogi wisdom

"Gaining mastery over my urge to devour squirrels has not been easy, but loving-kindness meditation helps me to control it." — Pi

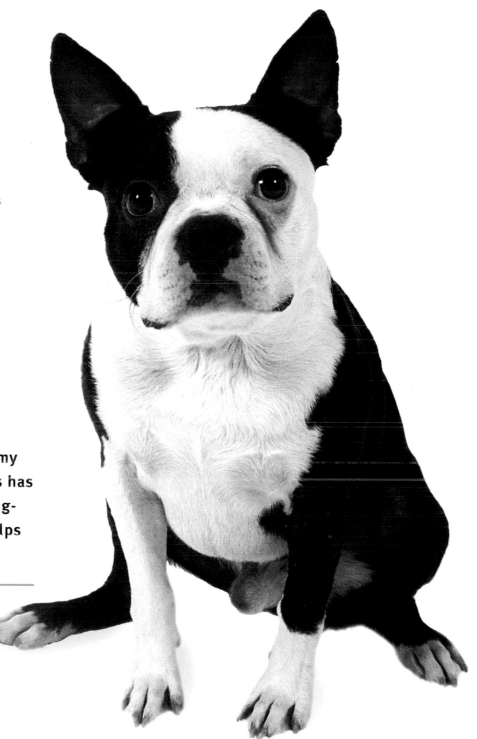

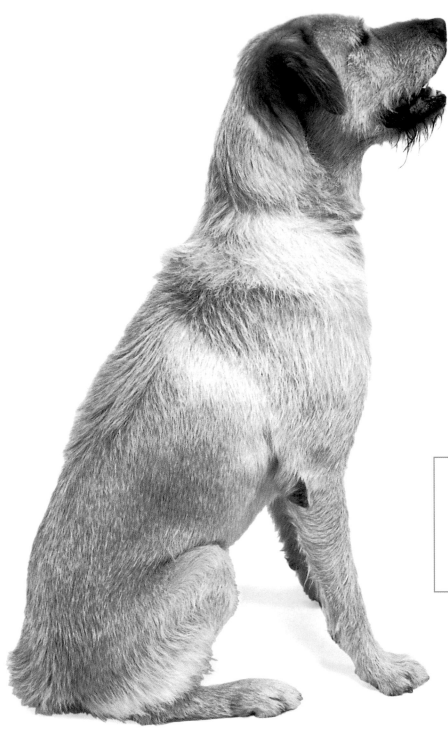

3 Buster practices an advanced meditation, concentrating on the image of his favorite bone. As he repeats the mantra, "bone, bone, bone," he calls to mind all of its aspects: its color, its smell, its taste, its texture, the feeling of it crunching between his teeth. Aware of his fierce desire for the bone, he is neverthe-less detached from this craving, able to focus on all its intricacies but not to act on it. This is a challenging meditation indeed.

human tip

Meditate with your dogi: sit together, breathe together, be in the moment together.

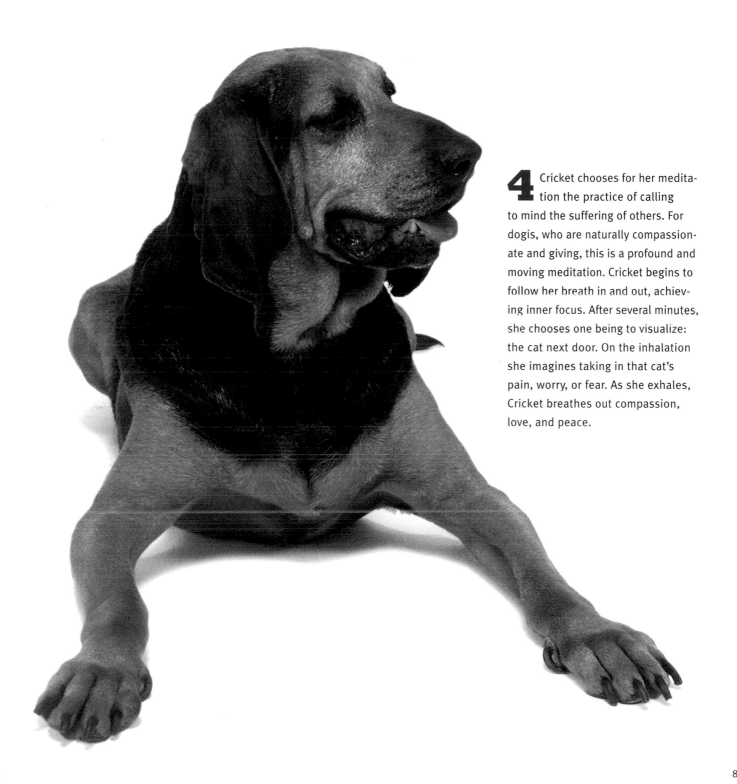

4 Cricket chooses for her meditation the practice of calling to mind the suffering of others. For dogis, who are naturally compassionate and giving, this is a profound and moving meditation. Cricket begins to follow her breath in and out, achieving inner focus. After several minutes, she chooses one being to visualize: the cat next door. On the inhalation she imagines taking in that cat's pain, worry, or fear. As she exhales, Cricket breathes out compassion, love, and peace.

closing chants

DOGIS TYPICALLY CHANT TO END THEIR PRACTICE AND ACKNOWLEDGE THEIR RENEWED SENSE OF ONENESS WITH THE UNIVERSE. THEY MAY CHANT OM, OR THEY MAY CHOOSE ANOTHER MANTRA THAT SUITS THEIR MOOD. WHEN DOGIS GET TOGETHER, THEY OFTEN DECIDE TO CHANT IN UNISON, A HARMONIC REMINDER OF HOW EVERYONE AND EVERYTHING IS CONNECTED.

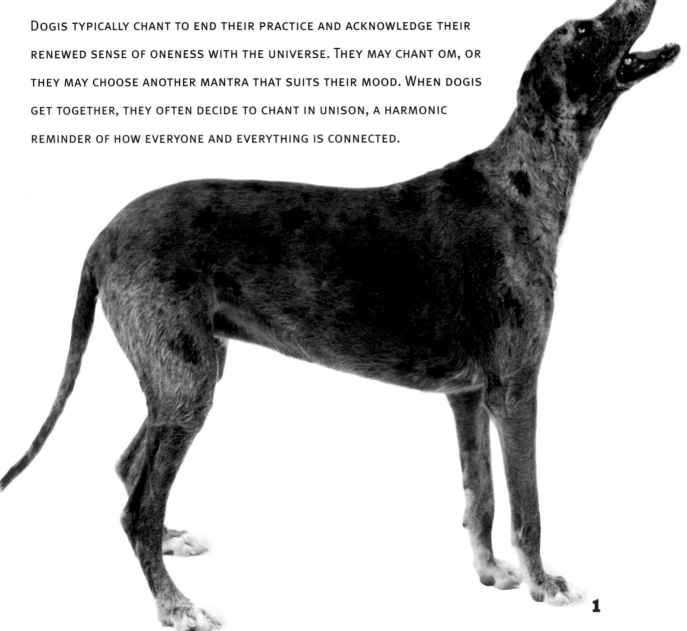

1

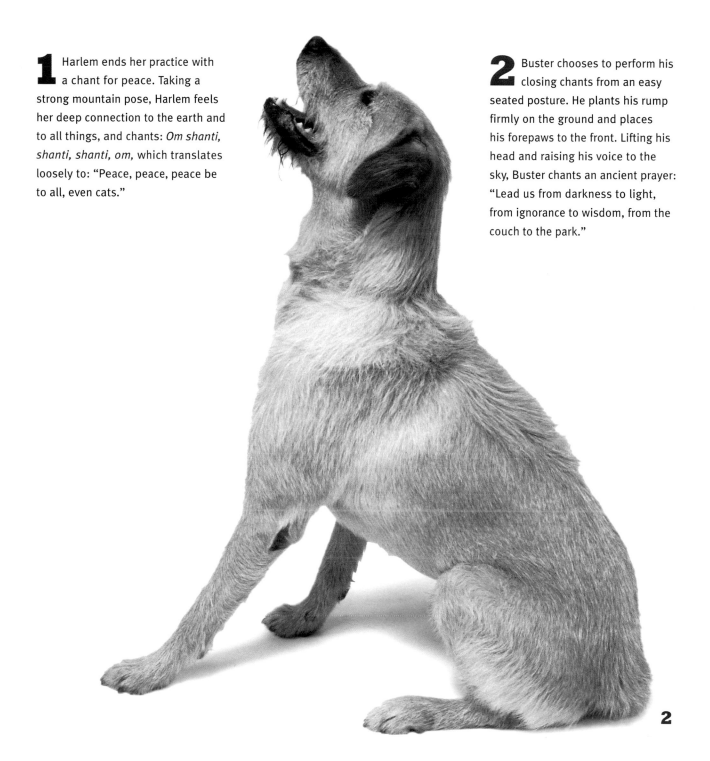

1 Harlem ends her practice with a chant for peace. Taking a strong mountain pose, Harlem feels her deep connection to the earth and to all things, and chants: *Om shanti, shanti, shanti, om,* which translates loosely to: "Peace, peace, peace be to all, even cats."

2 Buster chooses to perform his closing chants from an easy seated posture. He plants his rump firmly on the ground and places his forepaws to the front. Lifting his head and raising his voice to the sky, Buster chants an ancient prayer: "Lead us from darkness to light, from ignorance to wisdom, from the couch to the park."

2

index of asanas

ASANA	DOGI	PAGE
opening chants		10
breathing awareness		12
victorious breath		14
chin lock		16

ASANA	DOGI	PAGE
breath of fire		17
alternate-nostril breathing		20
cooling breath		21
mountain pose		22

ASANA	DOGI	PAGE
downward-facing dog		24
upward-facing dog		30
upward-paw pose		32
chin, chest, knees		34

ASANA	DOGI	PAGE
chaturanga		36
jump		37
chair pose		38
warrior		40

ASANA	DOGI	PAGE
triangle pose	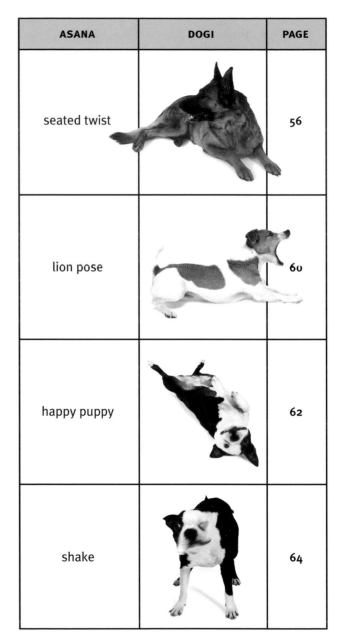	42
pup's pose		44
boat pose		48
cobra		50

ASANA	DOGI	PAGE
seated twist		56
lion pose		60
happy puppy		62
shake		64

ASANA	DOGI	PAGE
roll	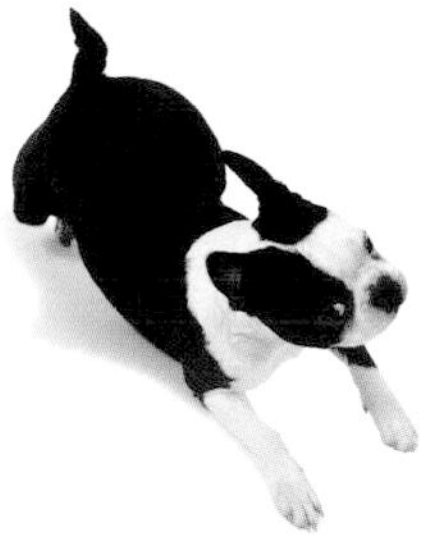	64
shoulder-opening poses	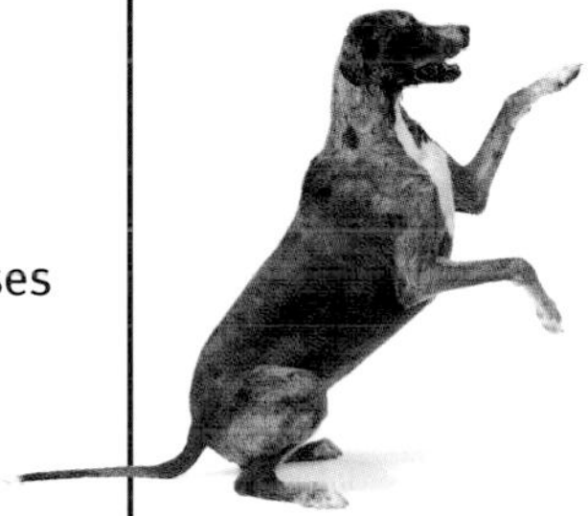	66
hip-opening poses	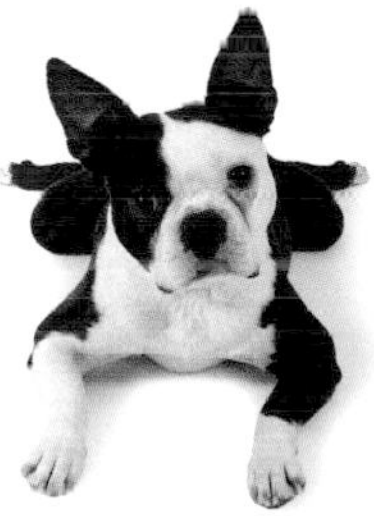	68
lotus pose	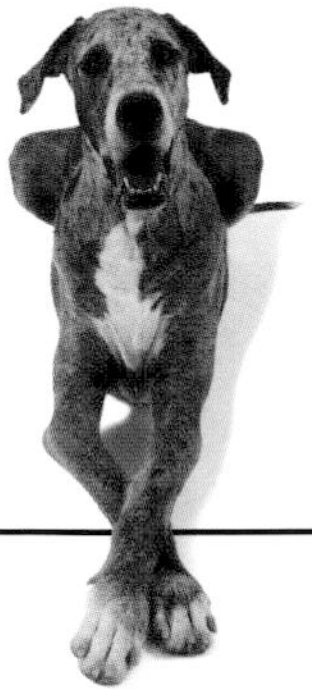	72

ASANA	DOGI	PAGE
corpse pose	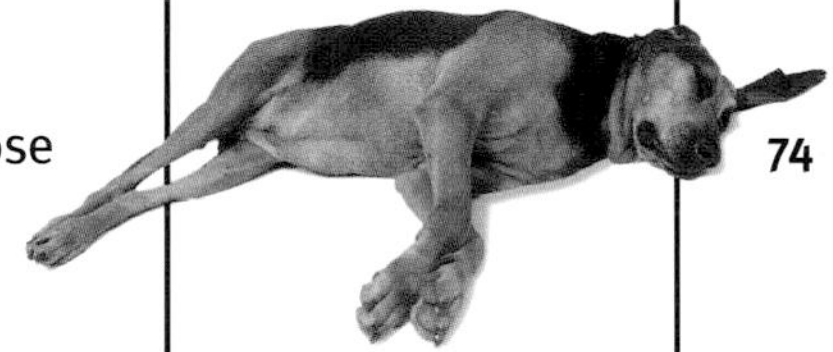	74
sense withdrawal	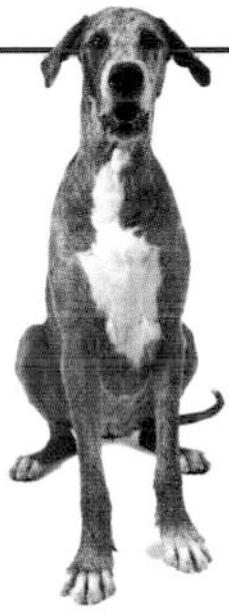	78
meditation	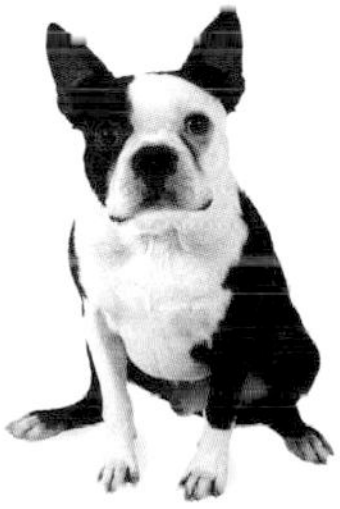	80
closing chants	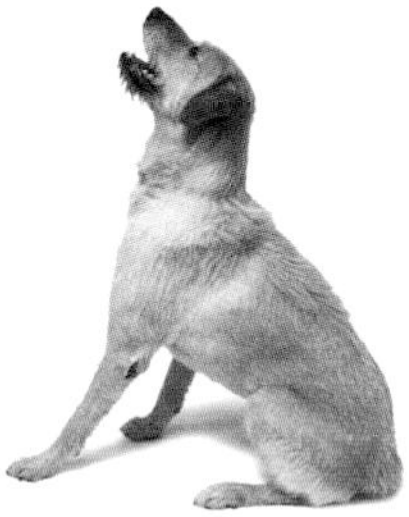	84

about the dogis

Bennie

Bennie is a Jack Russell terrier. He comes from a long line of dogis, and has studied doga under the revered teacher Paws Dogananda. In his practice, Bennie seeks to blend the physical challenges of "power" doga with the spiritual growth that allows the individual dogi to transcend his own experience and find unity with the universe. Bennie speaks frequently at doga conferences, and conducts workshops from his home base in East Hartford, Connecticut. His best-known workshop is "The Unity of Doga: Overcoming Hostility to Squirrels, Skunks, and Chipmunks."

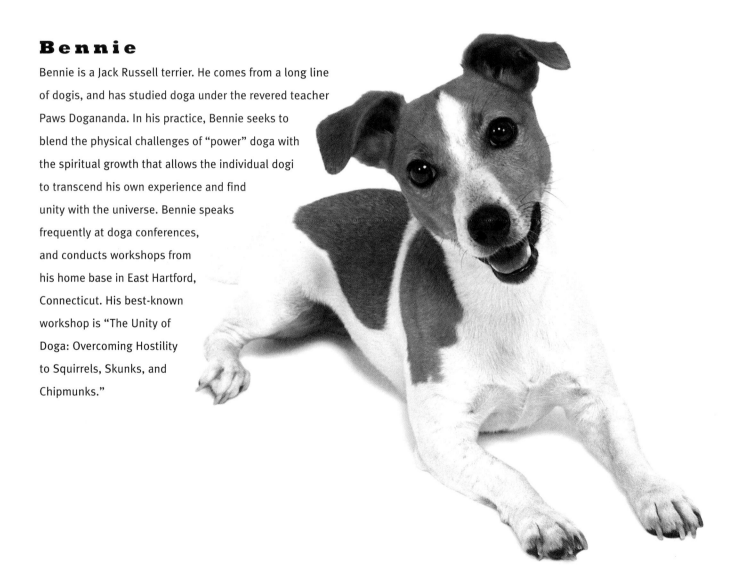

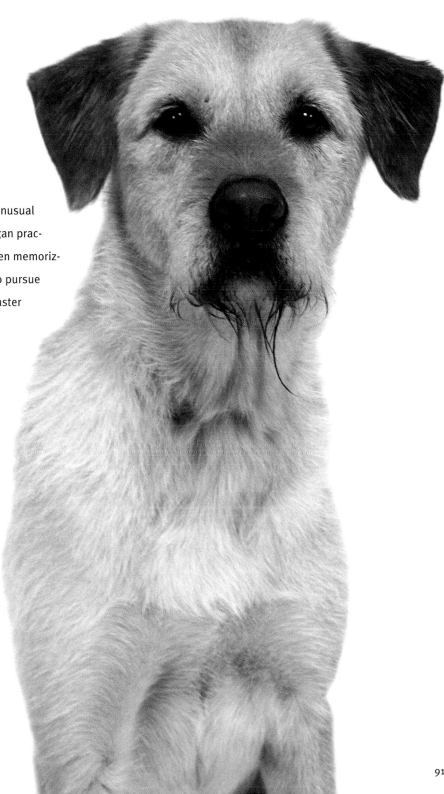

Buster

A terrier mix, Buster came to doga through an unusual
path. A well-known Broadway actor, he first began practicing doga techniques to improve his focus when memoriz-
ing roles. His improved concentration led him to pursue
further training, and he became a student of master
dogi Arfit Dogai. Buster focuses on the mind-
body connection in his practice, with particular
emphasis on breathing techniques. Buster
lives in Higganum, Connecticut, where he
cofounded the world's first doga studio with
fellow dogis Cricket and Pi. He is the author
of *Panting or Pranayama? Doga Breathing
for Beginners*.

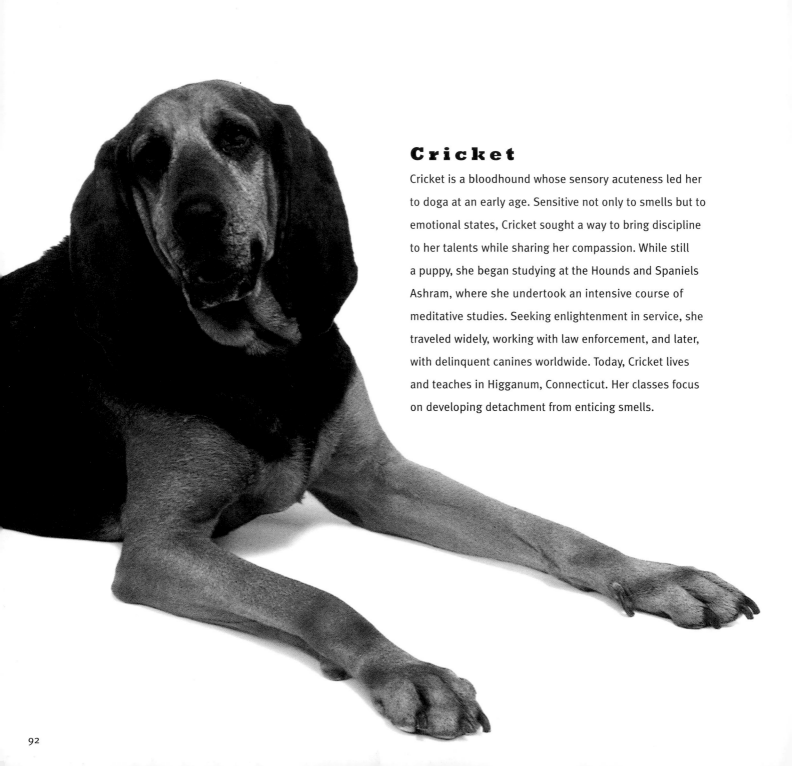

Cricket

Cricket is a bloodhound whose sensory acuteness led her to doga at an early age. Sensitive not only to smells but to emotional states, Cricket sought a way to bring discipline to her talents while sharing her compassion. While still a puppy, she began studying at the Hounds and Spaniels Ashram, where she undertook an intensive course of meditative studies. Seeking enlightenment in service, she traveled widely, working with law enforcement, and later, with delinquent canines worldwide. Today, Cricket lives and teaches in Higganum, Connecticut. Her classes focus on developing detachment from enticing smells.

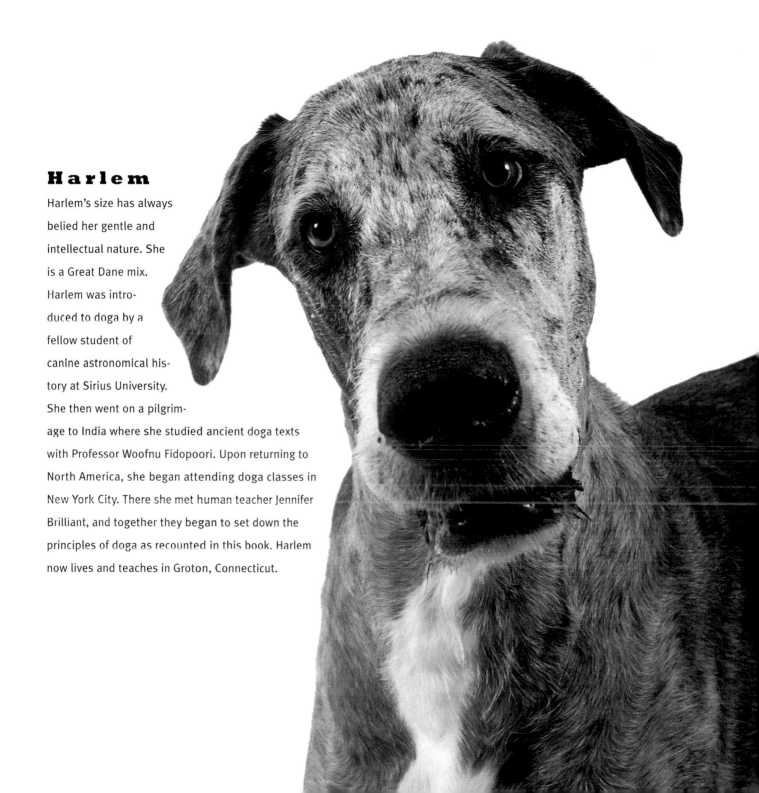

Harlem

Harlem's size has always belied her gentle and intellectual nature. She is a Great Dane mix. Harlem was introduced to doga by a fellow student of canIne astronomical history at Sirius University. She then went on a pilgrimage to India where she studied ancient doga texts with Professor Woofnu Fidopoori. Upon returning to North America, she began attending doga classes in New York City. There she met human teacher Jennifer Brilliant, and together they began to set down the principles of doga as recounted in this book. Harlem now lives and teaches in Groton, Connecticut.

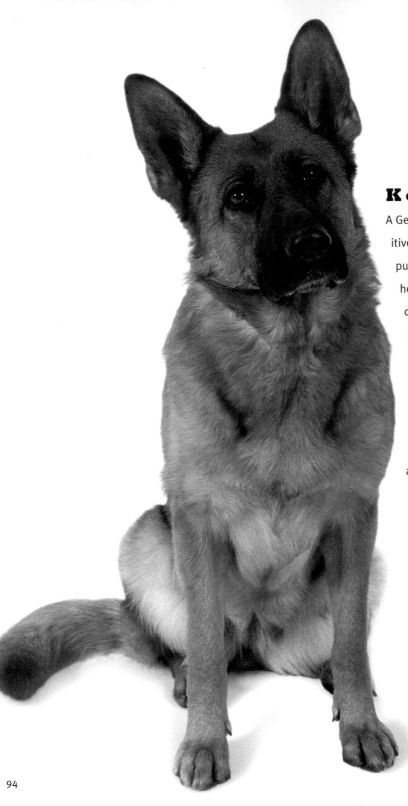

Kessie

A German shepherd, Kessie is a natural athlete and competitive frisbee player who came to doga as therapy for a pulled thigh muscle. She found that the practice improved her jumping and catching performance, and became a doga devotee. Kessie trained at the Dogaville Hatha Doga Academy, studying the various hatha styles until she arrived at a synthesis that suited her athletic inclinations. A new mother, her current focus is balancing mind, body, and spirit with the demands of six puppies. Kessie lives in Monson, Massachusetts, where she trains doga teachers, and offers pre-natal and parent-puppy doga classes.

Pi

Pi is a Boston terrier. Revered worldwide as a master dogi, Pi pioneered the Pupengar style of hatha doga in North America. He studied directly under Barkus Pupengar, and translated *The Pupengar Way* into Doggish. Pi has trained many doga teachers in the stillness of Pupengar, in which dogis learn to hold savasana for prolonged periods while mastering the breath. Often confused with sleeping, this prolonged savasana actually brings the dogis to a new plane of consciousness. As a result, dogis who train with Pi are distinguished by their ability to retain a gentle smile through the most challenging of situations and in all states of awareness. Pi lives in Higganum, Connecticut, where he works with Bill Berloni to introduce humans to doga.

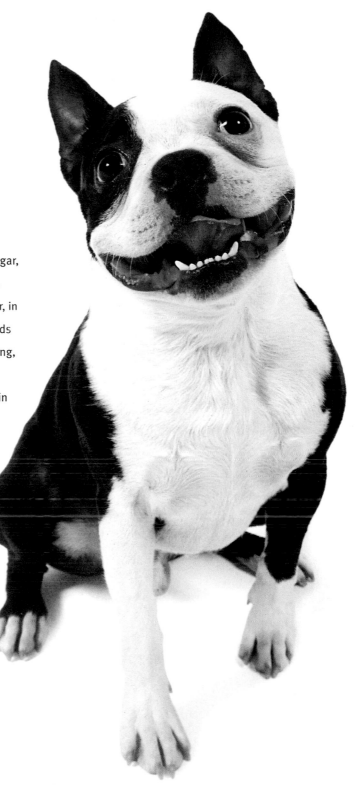

about the authors

Jennifer Brilliant

Jennifer Brilliant is the Director of Teacher Training at OM yoga center in New York City. In addition to teaching private and group classes, Jennifer also teaches special workshops for scoliosis as well as "Deepening Your Home Practice." She has 18 years of experience guiding people and dogs of all levels in athletic, therapeutic, and creative movement. Jennifer lives in Brooklyn, New York, with her husband, daughter, and dogi, Maxx.

My love and thanks to my husband, Jeff, for his unfailing support and his inspiring love of dogs, and to my friend Cyndi Lee, who has brought so many good things to my life. Thanks to Dr. Karen Mateyak, a true dogi guru, for helping and healing all dogs. —J.B.

William Berloni

William Berloni has been a professional animal trainer since 1976 and since then, his animals have performed in hundreds of films, commercials, television shows, printed work, and theater across North America. He runs his New York company, William Berloni Theatrical Animals, with his wife, Dorothy. He has won the ASPCA Humanitarian Award, the Capital Area Humane Society Humane Award, and the American Humane Association Richard Craven Award. William is also the behavior consultant for the Humane Society of New York. He personally trains Buster, Pi, and Cricket.

William would like to thank his trainers, Valerie Whiterock (Bennie), Fredericka Garreffa (Kessie), and Tammy Karecki (Harlem).